REALLY MANAGING

The Work of Effective
CEOs in Large
Health Organizations

AMERICAN COLLEGE OF HEALTHCARE EXECUTIVES
MANAGEMENT SERIES

Anthony R. Kovner, Series Editor

Anthony R. Kovner

REALLY MANAGING
The Work of Effective CEOs in Large Health Organizations

MANAGEMENT SERIES
American College of Healthcare Executives

Library of Congress Cataloging-in-Publication Data

Kovner, Anthony R.
   Really managing.

   1. Health services administration. 2. Health
services administrators—Interviews. I. Title.
RA971.K65   1988   362.1'068   88-2673
ISBN 0-910701-32-6

Health Administration Press
A Division of the Foundation of the
   American College of Healthcare Executives
1021 East Huron Street
Ann Arbor, Michigan 48104-9990
(313) 764-1380

*To my wife Chris, and to
my daughters Sarah and Anna.*

Contents

Preface

Large health care organizations are changing rapidly and face increased competition and risk of failure. We know little about what chief executive officers (CEOs) do or their contribution to organizational effectiveness. I have written elsewhere that CEOs must "assume more power and be held more accountable" if health care organizations are to survive and grow in today's competitive environment (Kovner 1985, 4). Here I suggest that we must understand better what CEOs do in order to evaluate their performance.

This book is divided into three parts. In Part One I discuss the conceptual and experiential frameworks and the design of the study. In Part Two I present interviews with four CEOs and their close associates, and I indicate the activities and episodes of work I observed when following the CEOs.

In Part Three I extract from the data four themes common to managerial effectiveness in large health care organizations, and I recommend actions managers can take relative to these crosscutting themes. Finally, I examine the usefulness of activities and episodes of work in evaluating managerial performance and make recommendations to managers regarding implementation of them.

Acknowledgments

Funding for the study upon which this book is based was provided generously by the Pew Memorial Trust. I wish to thank the four CEOs for graciously welcoming me into their organizations. I'm grateful to them and to Art Brief, John Griffith, Chris Kovner, Duncan Neuhauser, and Steve Shortell for their comments on an earlier paper which was the basis of this book. I deeply appreciate Blair Potter's editorial assistance in improving the quality of my writing. I also thank Lisa Buneo, who spent many days helping to produce a finished manuscript.

Anthony R. Kovner
October 1987

Abbreviations

AIDS	acquired immune deficiency syndrome
CCU	coronary care unit
CEO	chief executive officer
CFO	chief financial officer
COO	chief operating officer
CT	computerized tomography
DRG	diagnosis-related group
ER	emergency room
HMO	health maintenance organization
IPA	independent practice association
JCAH	Joint Commission on Accreditation of Hospitals (now the Joint Commission on Accreditation of Healthcare Organizations)
M.B.A.	master of business administration
M.D.	doctor of medicine
MRI	magnetic resonance imaging
NHC	neighborhood health center
NIH	National Institutes of Health
OB-GYN	obstetrics-gynecology
OEO	Office of Economic Opportunity
PPO	preferred provider organization
PR	public relations
VIP	very important person
VP	vice-president

Part One

Frameworks and Study Design

The desire to verify conjecture, to witness spontaneous, unstructured events in the wild, is of course very sharp among field biologists. Nothing—no laboratory result or field-camp speculation—can replace the rich, complex texture, the credibility, of something that took place "out there." And scientists working in the field know that what they see in the field always has the potential to contradict what they have read or been told. One-time events, like seeing a polar bear stalk and kill a seal in open water, may be of no statistical importance. It may not be possible, in other words, to generalize about all bears from these incidents. But such events emphasize the resourcefulness of the individual bear and the range of capability in the species; or they may reveal an unusual technique widespread only in a certain population. These events underscore something critical in the biology of large predators: the range of capability in the species. No matter how long you watch, you will not see all it can do.

—Barry Lopez, 1986

1.

Conceptual Framework

By "conceptual framework" I mean my intellectual sources and my background of practical experience, which necessarily bias my views on health care management. I wrote my doctoral thesis on the organization of eight hospital nursing units. How are nursing units with different technologies staffed in the hospital? How should they be staffed? My subsequent research has been primarily on hospital governance. Are hospital boards organized to make effective policy decisions? Are trustees selected for their capability and experience in making such decisions? I have also examined the participation of physician leaders in strategic planning in hospitals (Kovner and Chin 1985). To what extent does this participation differ with organizational circumstances and hospital size and complexity?

In this book, I present a study of managerial work in four large health care organizations. The concepts I have found most useful are episodes of work, managerial choice, the leadership challenge, and specifying of objectives.

Activities and Episodes of Work

One of my key themes in analyzing what managers do is the usefulness of the concepts of activities and episodes of managerial work. Strauss

et al. (1985) have written about the organization of medical work for patients with chronic illness and its impact on those who do the work. The
authors describe the contingencies that workers cannot control (in part
because the patient is part of the work process) and the difficulties of
managing chronic illness, including the longer-than-usual care trajectory
and the importance of care rather than disease management.

In managing chronic care, practitioners shape rather than control the
work, which they experience emotionally. In diagnosing problems, the
providers of care estimate the potential course of the illness without medical intervention. Then they map what the interventions might be, what
might happen if the interventions are effective, what resources are required to make the interventions, and the patient's location along the
course of the disease, which is a judgment call.

In organizing therapeutic action, providers generate a search for options of treatment, because many chronically ill patients are defined as
"problematic." Unexpected contingencies occur. Operational decisions
are made to get the trajectory into the best manageable order. It is not
always a simple matter to say who is in charge. Specialists share in the
shaping of the work. There are debates over trajectory. Clusters and se-
quences of tasks constitute the details of trajectory work (Strauss et al.
1985).

There are many implications for managing large health care organizations. The work involves dealing with contingencies that managers cannot control, managing others who are part of the management process
itself, and episodes or projects that take a long time to accomplish mean-
ingful results. Managers estimate early on what would happen without
management intervention. Operational changes must be made midcourse
in order to adjust work flow. It is not always a simple matter to say who
is in charge. Specialists share in the shaping of the work to be done.
There are debates over what should be done and how. Clusters and se-
quences of tasks constitute the details of managerial work.

Managerial Choice

Brown writes about the organizational cost to health maintenance
organizations (HMOs) of their mission of comprehensiveness and responsibility (1983). Management of HMOs demands coordination of highly
diverse substantive tasks with different technologies; the HMO combines
in one structure a collegium of professionals—highly trained scientists
delivering intimate human services—and a business that is competitive,
entrepreneurial, and preoccupied with the bottom line. Conflicts arise
easily and are difficult to resolve. There is great organizational fragility.

Managers must constantly make trade-offs all across the economic and political spheres and between short-term and long-term benefits.

Brown argues that managers must design the optimum size and location of facilities and number and specialty mix of staff in light of actual, expected, or desired membership. It is difficult to find managers who have specialized skills, knowledge of local conditions and attitudes, and negotiating ability in addition to an ability to get along well with employees and other contributors. Management skills and experience must change as an HMO grows larger and more complex, and the early, valued images of organizational character may get in the way of dynamic growth (Brown 1983).

Implications of Brown's analysis are that managers in large health care organizations are constantly making choices, not so much regarding policy as use of their time, given the overwhelming abundance of stimuli and the complexity of the managerial field. Although a large part of the CEO's job may be making policy decisions, it is in the formulation and implementation of such decisions that managers make daily and strategic choices.

The Leadership Challenge

Kotter writes that diversity and interdependence are characteristic of large modern organizations (Kotter 1985). There are differences among workers with respect to goals, values, stakes, assumptions, and perceptions. Interdependence exists among parties who have power over each other because they are to some degree dependent on each other. Managers must get others to help and cooperate, but they often do not have control over those others. More and more jobs in large organizations have a built-in gap between the power one needs to get the job done well and the power that automatically comes with the job.

Managerial power is derived from information or knowledge, good working relationships, personal skills, intelligent agendas for action, resource networks (through which agendas are implemented), and good track records in managing. Skillful managers develop the power sources they need to create effective agendas and networks. This is not easy: It requires time, effort, and constant attention (Kotter 1985).

Large health care organizations, in particular, suffer from these built-in gaps between responsibility and authority. They are characterized by so much diversity and interdependence that perhaps more of them should be reorganized into smaller entities with some centralized control but without centralized management. How do health care managers build appropriate agendas and develop resource networks? What does this mean for the structuring of the CEO position in large health care organizations? These are subjects about which little has been written.

Specifying Objectives

Hales defines effectiveness as the extent to which what managers actually do matches what they are supposed to do (1986). He summarizes what is known about managerial work as follows:

—It combines a specialist-professional element and a general managerial element

—The substantive elements involve essentially liaison, human-management, and responsibility for a work process

—The character of work elements varies by duration, time span, recurrence, unexpectedness, and source

—Much time is spent in day-to-day trouble-shooting and ad hoc problems of organization and regulation

—Much managerial activity consists of asking or persuading others to do things, involving the manager in face-to-face verbal communication of limited duration

—Patterns of communication vary in terms of what the communication is about and with whom the communication is made

—Little time is spent on any one activity, particularly on the conscious, systematic formulation of plans

—Managers spend a lot of time accounting for and explaining what they do, in informal relationships and in politicking

—Managerial activities are riven by contradiction, crosspressures, and conflicts; much managerial work involves coping with and reconciling social and technical conflicts

—There is considerable choice of what is done; part of managerial work is setting the boundaries of and negotiating the work itself.

There is no clear standard in terms of what others expect or require managers to do (Hales 1986).

Perhaps because of the lack of agreement as to what health care encompasses, how best to produce it, and what the goals of large health care organizations ought to be, these organizations are characterized by a lack of objectives against which a manager's contribution can be measured. The difficulty of isolating a manager's contribution to goal attainment in these organizations further complicates matters. As the health care industry becomes more competitive, specifying measurable organizational objectives will be increasingly critical to obtaining and retaining market share—as will evaluating managers' use of time in attaining those objectives.

2.

Experiential Framework

I have spent 12 years managing health care organizations and a similar amount of time teaching about their management. My first job in health care was managing a 60-bed nursing home. After five years of work on my master's and doctoral degrees, I became assistant administrator of a 500-bed not-for-profit hospital; soon thereafter I was promoted to administrator of a large ambulatory care center managed by the same not-for-profit hospital under contract to the New York City government.

My next position was group practice manager in a department of medicine at an academic health center in Philadelphia. I later became director of a program in health care administration at the University of Pennsylvania. I went to Detroit as senior health consultant for the United Auto Workers. Subsequently, I became chief executive officer of a 215-bed not-for-profit hospital in southern New Jersey.

Currently I am director of the graduate program in health policy and management at New York University's Graduate School of Public Administration. In my teaching I emphasize the art and politics of management and case studies rather than management science and the application of quantitative methods.

For several years I have spent about one-third of my time managing two rural hospital demonstration programs for The Robert Wood Johnson Foundation. I have also consulted for several large health care organizations and have been a trustee of other large health care organizations.

3.

Study Design

This exploratory study was carried out between January and July 1986 in four large health care organizations in the northeast United States. For my six months of sabbatical leave, I chose a project that I felt was doable and important. "Doable" meant that the number of sites and their geographical locations would necessarily be constrained. During the life of the study, nine CEOs were considered for observation. My preference was for CEOs with five or more years' job tenure in health care organizations with annual sales of $75 million or more. I also wanted institutions that were in different circumstances. I had considered contrasting effective and ineffective CEOs, but I rejected the idea because of the difficulties this would pose in gaining access to the CEOs and in publishing the results.

The selection process used was to ask CEOs, one by one, to participate, until the desired number of four was reached. Five CEOs who were asked did *not* participate in the study: one resigned to run for political office, two were fired, and two declined. That two of the CEOs I chose were subsequently fired may raise questions about my perceptions of effectiveness. I would respond that effective CEOs have been fired—and more than once. I do not claim that these four chosen *are* effective CEOs, only that they are CEOs of large health care organizations who have held their positions for a number of years and that I believe them to be effective.

The four participating CEOs have been in their present positions for five years or more and work in large not-for-profit health care organizations with gross revenues in 1984 of $85 million or more and with 500 employees or more.

Prior to the study I knew three of the nine CEOs very well, two slightly, and four not at all. Of the four CEOs who participated, I knew two well and the other two by reputation. My beliefs as to the effectiveness of the nine CEOs were based upon the following: my perceptions of their local reputation (this was not systematically derived, but I did ask others about the CEOs whom I did not know well); the size and perceived achievement of their institutions relative to others in the area; and their longevity in their jobs, which is unusual in large health care organizations.

After a preliminary meeting, I interviewed each of the four CEOs twice, for a total of three hours. The questions I asked them are shown in Appendix A. Several of the questions were adopted from Levinson and Rosenthal (1984, 292–94). About 90 percent of the two interviews is presented in narrative form in Chapter 4. These narratives were edited and subsequently reviewed by the CEOs for accuracy.

As part of the study, each CEO was asked for the names of eight or nine close associates who had direct experience with his work. I interviewed each of these 34 individuals for 60 to 75 minutes. Interviews with four associates of each CEO are presented in Chapter 5, also in narrative form. This selection was made to avoid repetition. About 80 percent of the 16 interviews is presented. The questions asked each interviewee are listed in Appendix B. The positions held by all 34 people interviewed are shown in Table 3.1.

Obviously, allowing the CEOs to choose the persons to be interviewed introduces a bias. I asked to speak with close associates representing a range of occupations, inside and outside the health care

Table 3.1: Positions Held by Interviewees

Position	All Interviewees	Those Reported Here
Associate, assistant administrator	10	6
Clinical chief, manager of clinical center	8	5
Chairman of the board, board members	4	2
Chief operating officer	4	1
Chief executive officer of another organization	2	0
Chief financial officer	2	2
Other*	5	0
Total	35	16

*Hospital association president, auditor, attorney, executive, secretary, and ex-wife. Those interviewed who were not employed by the CEO's present organization totaled six: hospital association president, auditor, attorney, ex-wife, and the medical director and two CEOs of other organizations.

organization. I specifically wished to include trustees, other managers, and physician leaders. Close associates were not entirely laudatory of the CEOs with whom they worked, but all of them believed their CEO to be effective, although not in every aspect of the job.

Between the two interviews, I followed each CEO for five consecutive days during a week of his choice. One CEO had to be out of town unexpectedly for a day, so I spent one day of the next week with him instead. In every case, I spent most of each long working day with the CEO. There were some confidential meetings and some other meetings after work that I did not attend, but every CEO said he reported to me what these meetings were about and with whom they were held. In the cases of two of the CEOs, there were no confidential meetings during working hours from which I was excluded. Three days of following are summarized for each CEO in Chapter 6. In addition, for each CEO, activities surrounding one episode that extended over the three days of following are abstracted.

I also reviewed annual reports, articles written by or about the CEO and the organization, and financial analyses of all four organizations. I took copious but not verbatim notes during the interviews and observations; I did not use a tape recorder. I summarized the data daily and had all my notes typed to facilitate analysis. I then summarized the data and isolated themes.

Part Two

Empirical Findings

*You operate constantly not knowing who your
customer is—is it the employer, who adds
costs to his product by adding health services;
the patient, who expects everyone to be
friendly and nice; the physician, who wants the
latest equipment and the most supportive
nurses; labor unions, who throw their entire
aspirations regarding career development,
salary, and professional prestige in the CEO's
lap? The CEO has to deliver. At any moment,
night or day, the slightest procedural mistake
can harm a patient.*

—Hospital chief operating officer,
Spring 1986

4.

Interviews with CEOs

Four CEOs were interviewed on two occasions about their work and what makes them effective. To preserve anonymity, they and their organizations are given fictitious names. For continuity and ease of reading, the interview questions (Appendix A) have not been repeated, the two interviews have been combined, and the CEOs' responses have been slightly edited. This was done primarily by omitting responses to questions 10 and 11 for the first interview and to question 17 for the second interview for all four CEOs.

Tim George, CEO of Washington Medical Center

Background

Washington Medical Center has over 1,000 beds, more than 5,000 employees, and gross annual revenues of over $300 million. It is part of an academic health center with more than 2,000 faculty members and has a mission of excellence in teaching, research, and service. Technology and mission are complex at Washington Medical Center, and the hospital is therefore less susceptible to being centrally managed. Because of its

ample resources and strong reputation, Washington Medical Center is
believed to face relatively little threat to operating finances or market
share.

Tim George is 64 years old, was educated as a physician, has worked
at the medical center for more than 30 years, and has been in his present
position for more than 15 years. He was interviewed on January 20, 1985,
and May 20, 1986.

Interview

My job immediately before being appointed CEO was as acting
chairman of a department. I viewed the hospital as a place where we
took care of a lot of sick patients, educated medical staff and house
officers, and conducted clinical experiments—an academic setting in
which we took care of our patients. Any institution at any time has
strengths and weaknesses. Some clinical departments are on the up-
swing or downswing, so you look at the ones which aren't doing so
well and try to improve the situation with the chairman or get a replacement. We had a lot of changes in department chairmanships
when I came into the job. In consultation with the dean [of the medical school], I was heavily involved in recruiting, providing support
for, and launching new chairmen. The most important things you do
in this job are recruiting chairmen and assisting them in recruitment.
I think the dean would say the same thing. It sets the tone, and if we
make a mistake, we suffer for it for a long time.

The board didn't give me a specific charge. These issues I've been
talking about emerged in our discussions. The members felt I had
lived in this kind of environment and in this specific academic health
center long enough to have a basis for my opinions on strengths and
weaknesses. So they were comfortable in having a nonbusiness leader
for the hospital. I don't recall what they said about financial affairs.
The assumption was that the hospital would run modest deficits—it
always had because of the free care it provides. They hoped the financial situation would improve but not at the expense of the mission
of the hospital. The bottom line had never been positive and wouldn't
be so long as we provided free care. We have sufficient income from
gifts and endowments to cover the operating losses. We were not
eroding principal, but we were not building it through operations
either. We have never had a year when the net-net was in the red.

I approached the job with the idea that our institution would be
one of the best. I thought the hospital was one of the best and I
intended for it to stay that way. You can't prove that you are number
one or number two, so why get hung up on it? Most of the evaluations

of the "best" hospitals are done by mass circulation magazines. But there is a sense as to which are the best institutions. You get a feel for it. At the medical school there are more quantitative measures for assessment than at the hospital—How many NIH grants did you bring in? For how much? For the hospital you can't use crude measures like the mortality rate. You sense quality from communications with peers. You can't ignore beauty magazines, but I don't take them seriously. We've always been on their lists, which keeps me from having to answer a lot of questions.

The weakness in measuring lies in the hospital's primary mission, taking care of patients. It's difficult to say patient care is better in one institution or another. The indices are too crude. Rates must be adjusted for case mix. Other indicators tend to be in the educational framework, the house staff we recruit. You know—of those you wanted to recruit, which ones did you get? I pay a lot of attention to that, and I go over this with the chiefs after the matching results come out. I ask, What's your reading of the performance? not, Did we get the top 10? They tell me what the last ranking was of the 10 we got (for example, number 30). Did the 10 choices fall between 1 and 10 except for one, or between 20 and 30? If so, where did the first 10 go? If the result was not as good as I would have liked, I ask the head of the department what we need to do to improve the situation. It may result from the experience that house staff have here—they can either get the appropriate experience at this hospital or rotate elsewhere. There may be a lack of leadership in the house staff program. Are we keeping in touch with our peer institutions to get the right kind of interest at the medical-school level? Do we need more elective programs? Are we getting students in to see the place early enough? There is an enormous grapevine among medical students, and these things change from time to time.

We've had to face the problem of our location. Primarily, I think, there is the perception that we only take care of rich people. Students are surprised that we have a substantial number of the same kinds of patients who are found at [public institutions]—we have a substantial clinic and ER patient population. Resident recruitment is all done by the departments. How much time do the departments spend on this process? They spend a lot of time on it, deservedly so. They are up front if they are disappointed, and we can usually agree upon what's missing—it's usually not too mysterious. [This city] is both an advantage and a disadvantage. Some love it here because they want to be part of the scene. Others don't want to put up with the hassle. My impression is that more look upon it as an advantage, and that's a change from when there was a negative image of the city.

This place, like most medical centers, is organized departmentally, so whenever you ask specifically about objectives, you get into departmental review and objectives. [A chairman of the hospital board] told new business types on the board, "This isn't the same as your business, and you don't do things the same way." I wasn't there, but my guess is that he was saying it's a much more collegial relationship—you must work with the chiefs to develop objectives that are consistent with institutional objectives but uniquely tailored to the needs of the departments. The department chairmen are ignorant of what their colleagues are up to.

It took me a while to sense the individuality of each of the departments. I knew a lot of the players, but I had to learn a lot. I knew the institution, so I didn't find the departments were doing something that came as a jolt; rather, I was learning the details of how they operated. The chiefs' objectives weren't out of line, they just didn't know the objectives of their colleagues. That's one of the things we have attempted to change by developing institutional objectives. We bring all the departments together and summarize plans and objectives for each other. This is not done on a scheduled basis, but periodically, when there's enough change to merit it. It was last done five years ago. We're updating plans now and will bring the chiefs together again.

The biggest change has been the effort to organize planning in a more systematic and orderly way. This is done in conjunction with the medical school, so it's an across-the-board plan—for patient care and for academic activities as well. (I was chairman of the planning committee—I've been here longer than the dean.) Before, there was no organized approach to planning. With our financial concerns (reimbursement and cutting back of research) we had to be more detailed and sophisticated. We set up a planning office and hired consultants. We involved faculty and staff in a detailed and lengthy procedure, probably because we hadn't done it before. We also did a detailed financial plan. We completed that plan about five years ago. The broad outlines haven't changed, but the details have, which is why we are redoing it. Results have been reassuring up to this point, but change is taking place more rapidly now.

There were three important aspects of the plan. First, we had to convince those who work here that the planning venture was important. There was a great deal of skepticism that there was any point to this; the planning exercise was bureaucratic and a waste of time. Gradually they began to realize there was something to be gained. They saw it best in dealing with their own departments, setting objectives and making plans to meet the objectives. There is less trouble now in talking to departments about this. They need staff help but not prodding. Second, the plan reaffirmed the overall hospital mission, which everyone agrees is to provide high-quality patient care, education, and research. This has to be reaffirmed and thought through. Should we place equal emphasis on these three aspects or not? After considering the alternatives, we came down with equal emphasis. This was an important decision, and it was made at all levels. It was especially important for the dean and hospital director. Such a mission required that neither emphasize one of these areas over the others.

Third, we had, for the first time in an organized fashion, plans for each clinical department. That, plus the overall institutional goals, permitted us to work out a strategy for implementing the plans, setting up a timetable for carrying out the plans, setting priorities in terms of what to do in what sequence, and devising a financial strategy for achieving them. Planning anything beyond five years is iffy, but we laid it out for ten years to accomplish the objectives. It's been important for us in our fund-raising efforts. These would otherwise be unguided, and if people are left to their own devices you can get into some awkward situations. Mrs. Jones may have different priorities in fund giving, so what do you do with her if she wants to give us money? We must keep bringing out our priority list and timetable for those raising money.

Ask other people [about my job]—and I'm not sure I want to hear the answers. It's a matter of style as much as anything. I've never lived in any other environment; I very much believe in the collegial approach to whatever we're doing. I have an open-door policy. People come in and talk about whatever is on their minds. I wander around to people's offices and in the hospital to see what's going on and to talk to people. I have certain set routines in terms of meetings, but I try not to have my time filled up that way. I have one- to one-and-a-half-hour meetings weekly with the administrative staff. The rest are individual and unplanned meetings. I don't like it when secretaries fill up my calendar with assigned appointments. I want to do things on the spur of the moment and for others to wander into my office. I don't know if they like it, but they get used to it. For example, I don't like to go to all the Christmas parties (there're so many of them), but I do. They know that I show up only briefly, but they'd know if I didn't show up too. It's important to greet all and wish them well. Big as we are, there is a remarkable family feeling here. The floor cleaners talk to me and address me; they feel it's okay, and that's how I want them to feel. I don't know how you can take care of patients in any other way. Everyone in the hospital should feel they're doing the same thing, taking care of the patient. If we are collegial, the patient will benefit. You've got to get out of your office. You can't allow shuffling papers and answering the phone, which is easy to keep doing in this business, to take over.

Being effective means being in contact broadly with the people who work here, having a feeling of family and a collegial approach to caring for patients. Not everyone has the same idea of how to do things. If an individual's approach is getting good results, you tolerate it because it works. If not, you've got to get it changed. I also do not believe in making end runs—if someone is not performing, I tell his or her supervisor what I have encountered and get the supervisor to fix it. I want everyone to be collegial, but there has to be organization. People hear from me if they try to make an end run around me.

The CEO must be aware of the external environment and anticipate changes that must be made. I spend a lot of time outside the institution. I have to be outside a good deal to sense what's going on in the environment and bring it back to the institution. I try to be involved in activities which give me early warning, such as hospital associations—local, state, and federal. They bring in legislative people. I spend one-third of my time outside the institution or on outside matters.

Take as an example HMOs, which are big and moving rapidly. We didn't rely only on our own personnel, we got a consulting firm in to assist us in dealing with managed care. We're still working on it. Each of us in administration is learning about managed care and seeing how other institutions are reacting—managed care has great significance for us. You have to go out there and talk with others facing the same problems and prospects. We keep the departments informed; a departmental task force of nonchairmen is following this along. When we have meetings with the chiefs, we go over what the task force is doing and significant events. My concern is that it's difficult to get to all the physicians fast enough. Communications from the chiefs down to attendings isn't fast enough.

Personnel decisions are the toughest. People are the most important thing you're dealing with, and your decisions will have an impact on the hospital. People are not inanimate things; you must be concerned with how they are affected. It's toughest when somebody is not doing the job and remedial approaches haven't worked. It's the worst part of the job.

It's happened with a department chairman—then I share that grief with the dean. Who is dean affects this job a lot. In dealing with clinical departments, anything of significance to the hospital is of significance to the dean too. We must reach agreement on whether it should be supported, how much, and by whom. We have two scheduled meetings a week and many conversations in between. We tend to divide where the meetings take place for symbolic reasons.

[The present] dean was prepared to be a dean, and he knew how faculty think who don't like administration. Deans have a lot of frustration, but he's doing the job and doing it well. He's reasonably tolerant of the faculty and their whims. We get along, although we don't always agree because we look at things differently. Medical schools live in a timeless world, while hospitals must respond to crises.

In this job you have to listen a lot to what the chiefs are talking about. It's a mistake to think you will direct these people. You can influence them, but you don't tell them, This is what you're going to do. If the chairmen turn against the guy in this job, he's finished. They're more likely to get him than governing boards, which are more tolerant. You must exert your influence indirectly. You must be working with them. A Harvard dean said, Make them think it's their idea. And it's true.

You also must address the concerns of the board. A few members lead it. Here, the board's concerns have been the same as the administration's. At times you see a different emphasis; you sometimes must play catch-up ball and address that. For example, we assumed that we had paid adequate attention to DRG reimbursement and had communicated this to the board. We then had to make an effort to tell the board in greater detail what we were doing. I did say that I didn't feel comfortable with the budget. We are preparing avidly for DRGs, but we aren't leading the board to believe that we can predict our budget with certainty. Board members have also been concerned with quality assurance. It's easy to overlook that issue in board meetings because we deal with it every day. They wanted to know how we keep tabs on our doctors, so we explained it to them. That may be more of a problem with an M.D. director—I may assume things because I am an M.D. that a non-M.D. would not assume. I do think we should have an M.D. as CEO here. Board members think that doctors are lousy businessmen. It's a widely held perception. I don't know if it's true. The most important aspects of this job have to do with quality of patient care and enough understanding of and participation in the academic side to ensure that it is held up as well. You must know qualities you're looking for and how to judge in recruiting. The physician familiar with academic medical centers is what is needed in this job.

We've been looking at succession planning. The corporate world is much better at this than we are; corporations figure it out for the next decade. We've been looking at who our backups are. I hope the result will be very able people down the line when I do leave this job. We need a spectrum of ages, too, so that not too many people leave at once.

Financial viability goes without saying. We've gone from a $40 million to a $300 million annual budget since I've been here. The hospital is financially sound; it has a good endowment by hospital standards; we still run an operating deficit which I'd love to get to break-even. We did it last year, but we won't this year or the next. We have enough nonoperating income to cover the deficit. We can take some degree of buffeting with all the changes, so I feel good about that—but I can't take credit for it.

To be an effective manager in the organization here, it is important that the individual have an academic medical center background, preferably as a physician. What distinguishes teaching hospitals is the inclusion of research and education with patient care. We have to educate medical students, residents, and technical personnel and do research and bring it to the bedside. That gives an individual who's grown up in that environment a real advantage. You must deal with clinical chiefs and subchiefs principally. You must talk to them on a peer basis. An academic physician doesn't need an interpreter.

The style that works best is a collegial one. You've got in front of you a constellation of departments and their heads. You don't hand down orders. You talk about problems. I carry that approach over to the nonprofessional side too. I try to solicit their views and am influenced by them. When you talk something through like that, the decision becomes apparent. Otherwise, you say, I think we heard from everybody; I'm going to put my vote in this direction; let's get on with it. Consensus is easier to reach than people think it is. If a clinical chief wants to do something new and different, we don't require other chiefs to approve. The problem with that is the others don't know what is going on. Communication becomes a problem. If one of my administrative department heads came forward, I would use the same approach. Frequently you forget to tell the other people.

When I came into this job, [evaluation] was strictly qualitative. I thought about it more in terms of patient care than business. Recently, because of the attitudes of the board president, we have a more quantitative assessment, one based on what we have projected. Now I would grade what I am doing in terms of how well we achieve those objectives. The advantage is that you have something quantitative to talk about. The disadvantage is that it doesn't allow for qualitative features, which are very important—they're the judgment call. I look at the quantitative factors, and I use the qualitative factors as adjustments. I make up an objectives statement for myself. I aggregate administrators' goal statements and include things that I think are particularly important. I found that my objectives were included in others', and I wanted to give them credit. What would happen if I went on sabbatical? It might make less difference than I might think. At some point the hospital would take a different tack because someone else who became dominant would emphasize different things. The CEO probably gets around more than anyone else so you have more observations to make on certain issues. Most everyone else spends most of their time inside.

The chief barriers [to managing effectively] relate to people. They don't all perform up to what you would like to see. Things don't get done with the speed and precision you'd hope for. It's not lack of resources. You've laid out things you thought were important, you thought the plan would be implemented, but it wasn't. Why not? You listen to the problems. Sometimes they're right. The objective was unrealistic or something unpredictable happened. You live with that or you make a change. At what point do you decide that you have to make a change, that your adjustments aren't working? These are usually well-motivated, loyal, well-meaning people. This makes it hard.

The opportunities [for managing effectively here] are more than you can cope with—pretty unlimited. The problem is you don't take the time to assess them and set priorities for them. You see an opportunity and jump at it. Only later do you recognize that you could have spent your time and resources better. But maybe you shouldn't worry about it too much or you wouldn't do as much. If something sounds good to me, my tendency is to say, Let's go! Nobody has unlimited resources—money, certificates-of-need—but that's relatively minor.

I probably wait too long to make necessary personnel changes. I hate to confront this type of decision and will procrastinate in a situation that is obvious, hoping for a miracle to occur. I may be a little too easygoing, not being emphatic when I feel emphatic about something, leaving my associates uncertain. Sometimes they say that— that they are unclear about where I stand or what I want.

I have become better able to assess and deal with a situation in a short period of time. That's experience! I have a feeling that in most situations that affect this hospital I can, in a brief period of time, assess accurately the significance of what I have observed and feel confident of what to do about it. It's a feeling I didn't have in the beginning. It's dangerous because it may not be justified and I may jump to conclusions that in the past I might have been more thoughtful about. A degree of inflexibility in approaching things can also develop, which is why someone maybe shouldn't stay in the job for 20 years. There are tremendous advantages to staying—you know the job—but maybe that keeps you from thinking generally or flexibly or creatively about what ought to be done.

We control costs in the budget process, set realistic targets and monitor them. If revenues are lower because occupancy is lower, we try to alter the expense side to bring it closer. If you don't want to cut quality or standards, there comes a limit, unless you're going broke. What I've learned from bitter experience is that, once you cut personnel, you run the risk of a snowball effect. This is particularly true in nursing. The others quit—There's no way we can carry that load—and they can get a job somewhere else.

The way we influence quality from this office is to constantly emphasize to the chiefs that quality is their primary responsibility at this hospital. What are they going to do about low performers? Prevention is most important. Don't bring anyone on the staff who hasn't been checked out carefully. That's why we tend to keep our own; we run the risk of inbreeding because we want known quantities. It's not a bad system. Actually, to call it inbreeding is not correct. There are two periods of mix and change: when students come to medical school and when interns are chosen.

Everyone thinks that what's coming will be different from what's happened. I don't know that that's so. Changes may be great, but not that different in terms of the challenges hospital directors confront. When I took this job, no one asked questions; you gave them the bill, and they made up the difference. That lasted three years. Then we got cost-containment regulations, which hit hard by the middle 1970s. That was a worse period than the present.

Larry Martin, CEO of Van Buren Hospital

Background

Van Buren Hospital has over 500 beds, more than 1,500 employees, and gross revenues of over $85 million. It is the smallest of the four observed organizations. Van Buren Hospital is believed to be lower in organizational complexity than the other organizations in the sample because it provides primary and secondary care only and does not emphasize the teaching or research mission. Van Buren provides a broad range of ambulatory care services in high volume and serves a low-income, as well as a middle-income, population. The hospital is believed to face a relatively stable environment because most of the residents in its two primary service areas receive hospital service at Van Buren and because most of Van Buren's services are provided to such residents.

Larry Martin is in his mid-fifties, has a master's degree in public health, and has been CEO for more than 15 years. He was interviewed on October 7, 1985, and May 19, 1986.

Interview

When I took over, Van Buren Hospital was a terrible loser. Everything that could be wrong was wrong. I asked myself, Could I have a personal impact? I didn't look like a candidate for a job like this— rather for the job of CEO in a major medical center. What's missing in that kind of job is the ability to have a dramatic personal impact— you spend most of your time tinkering. But if a strong person goes to a weak place, he or she could do something. The reputation [of Van Buren] was that the board interfered a lot. It has had a succession of administrators who couldn't cope.

I think the board hired me because they thought I was a good technician. I came from a nearby hospital which they thought highly of. They hoped [Van Buren] could be like it, stronger and more stable. They got that. I spent the better part of my first two years here doing what I had learned how to do as a technician in order to improve the operation.

What I got was a blank sheet from an institution that had run out of energy and ideas. That blank sheet allowed me to rewrite what the institution was. If you look at a speech that I made in 1970, you will see that I began by dealing with what a community service institution is, with health as well-being, with the hospital not simply as a group of patients but as an energetic and committed staff as well, with the hospital as a partner of the community, "us against the world." That's what I came for—to articulate a different view of what a place like this is, that it is not a physician's workshop. There was hardly anywhere I could go to do a thing like that—I couldn't have done it at [an academic medical center]. I have been trying to define a different kind of community hospital.

Everything had to be changed. [The staff's] attitude was defeatist: they knew they were going to lose every game. Their goal was to not embarrass themselves. I had to implant the notion that they could win, win, win. They lacked a proper sense of dignity. For example, the first day I walked in, I saw that the front entrance had a little plot of dirt on each side and a wrought iron fence. There was no grass there, and part of the fence was down with a pipe propping it up. I came in July and put sod in for instant grass and replaced the whole fence. It is important to realize that everyone walked in and out of the hospital yet had never seen what I saw. One of our senior M.D.'s liked the new entrance so much that he made a contribution covering the entire expense.

M.D.'s on the [Van Buren] staff had known me at the other hospital and said that I wasn't a bad person. I demanded a high salary, which equals respect. Then they pay attention to you. If you're paid average, they think you're average. After I finished the interview process and reached an understanding with the board that their behavior would change—they would stop overseeing everything and having crisis meetings—I said that I wanted to spend time with the medical leaders before saying yes. I did that. I told the medical leaders, "I want to interview you before I accept the job. I'll tell you what a hospital administrator is and how he relates to the medical staff. Now, I'm putting this appointment in your hands. If you don't want me to come, I won't come. This is the basic deal." I put it in their hands. Not only did the board think they had got someone they ordinarily couldn't have attracted, but the medical leadership had the sense that I had given them the power of appointing me and that I had a view of a very strong CEO.

Attitude is personal. I acted as if I knew what I was doing. I did things that had visibility. For example, I had some areas of the hospital painted. Van Buren had cost reimbursement then, and we couldn't raise capital to repair things. So we hired our own construction people, who would be reimbursable. All of a sudden, all kinds of work got done. The way you dress, the confidence with which you speak, are crucial to this whole thing. I am in the business of turning grays into blacks and whites, knowing that if I guess wrong often enough I'll get fired. I'm still doing that. I'm very careful about style. I shave before each board meeting. I arrange every detail of important meetings myself—the way the table is set up, for instance—everything should look right. You change attitudes that way.

At [Van Buren] we don't have policies in the real sense. I tell an honest, continuing story about what we're trying to do. We hold conversations in our board meetings about [Van Buren's] reason for being. The way policies are decided here is that I talk about our effort to serve our neighborhood—what we ought to do. I ask the board for support of me and of this philosophy. The members can speak up if they don't like it.

To change [Van Buren's] attitude, I did two things. First, I asked the city government to give us one of their hospitals. This is outside our area of services. It never worked out, but it showed I was trying to get something going. Second, we were aware of this three-acre property, and we put a few dollars down to hold it so we could consider rebuilding the hospital there. This was never a real possibility: there was no money and it was in the wrong neighborhood, but we created the impression that we were trying to change our situation. Then we came up with the idea of converting this building. We had the other property, and we were making interest payments on it. What were we going to do with it? I looked around and came up with senior citizen housing. I knew about the local community and the excessive number of aged. I found a mechanism to get our money on the property back and more, and at the same time to do a good thing for our neighborhood. I took my idea to the board, and everyone thought it was terrific. This is how we get our policies.

I can hardly believe the record myself. Almost everything we tried to do we did, with no money, no endowments, anything. We've created a very large, federally funded neighborhood health center.

Aside from improved housing, participation, and zoning, the basic health issues in our community were (1) lack of access to a physician delivery system, in one area, and (2) in an area with a rapidly aging, middle-class population served by fee-for-service practitioners, lack of a decent inpatient facility.

Being effective in my job means serving the neighborhood better. That's what I get paid for, I think. I am in a terrific position to convert resources for the neighborhood. The better I do that, the better I am at my work. I am this neighborhood's hospital administrator, not the doctors' or the trustees' administrator. I ask the trustees to see me in those terms. It used to be called community need, now it's called market demand. In those terms, we've penetrated and captured the market. People in the neighborhood receive their care through us, and this represents a substantial part of our business.

That doesn't mean that you don't need the confidence of the trustees and the medical staff or that you mustn't create an environment in which others can have fun and use their imaginations. I'm good at these things. People here are not only smart, they're nice people and have remained at Van Buren a long time. I think their stability has been important to our neighborhood.

The toughest decisions were all in the area of risk. The first NHC grant was for $785,000. We got the check, and we didn't have a thing— no space, no medical direction, no experience. If we failed with this— and you *can* fail—it would have been awful. We needed neighborhood participation that no one understood in those days. Second, we decided to convert this building into a modern hospital. No one in his right mind could have approved of that decision. Everything about this job was hard. The most difficult decision was taking the Van

Buren job and perhaps screwing up my career. All the odds were against success.

The major pitfall in this job is not knowing what you're doing. I thought it would be fun to redefine an institution, but I did know the nuts and bolts as a technician. You must also keep up with the way things work, such as changes in the reimbursement system. You can't get away with not knowing how the system works, and it takes a lot of time to keep up.

There is a fine line, in leadership, between being arrogant about your knowledge and work, and being arrogant toward people. As arrogant as I may appear about the details of my work, I apologize if I'm five minutes late. I do this all the time. You can't get to believing you know the work so well that you can forget common courtesy. As CEO, everyone treats you as special. It's okay so long as you don't believe you are special. Being CEO doesn't give you a right not to stand in the cafeteria line, or not to hold the elevator door for women waiting. They defer to you, but you must say *no* to such deference.

No matter who comes in next, it will be hard for that person to turn his or her back on this institution's promise to be responsive to the neighborhood—at least not in the short run. We've made it too many times in too many places. I do the best I can until the day I leave. After that day, I won't be able to get into the parking lot. I'm proud of the physical buildings and the idealistic definition of who we are. I also leave behind the sense that the CEO is really the key: he sets the style, attitude, and spirit, signals whether it is a risk-taking place or not, defines institutional choices. And I think that's good. Sometimes it goes too far—an institution can be too dependent on an individual—and I'm not sure how you balance that out. The right person gives the organization energy, honor, imagination—things only an individual can do. A board of 30 meeting once a month can't do that.

I wish I could make our hospital clinically more excellent. I'm not satisfied here. But we're doing as well as we can under the circumstances. Where we are is not considered a good place to serve by most physicians. This limits our attractiveness to the very top people in medicine. We can't be on the edge of new technology. We must wait until it becomes routine enough and the cost of having it moderate. To the extent that medical education attracts better physicians, we fail because we lack the resources to do medical education really right.

This is a tax-exempt institution. Others have forgotten what an incredibly idealistic thing a hospital is. A nearby hospital worries (in considering a merger with us) because we treat so many poor people.

They ought to be proud of us—it's the American thing to do. It's what the founders of this hospital said it should do when its doors were opened in the 1880s. No one knew what to do with poor people then. Rich people were treated at home. Taking care of the poor is in the hospital charter.

For example, it used to be that we didn't get automobile license plates by mail but had to go to the license bureau. I always did it at the last minute. I had to go at the end of February, and the office was set up in two storefronts. There was a long line when I got there. Inside was a counter and five clerks. There were three people standing in front of each clerk. Seventy-five people were standing outside. I asked the guard to let more people in. He said the clerks didn't like the noise and confusion. I said, I think *we* own this place and you don't. That's what the problem is. I believe that—the people we serve aren't a nuisance. It's easy to think in the hospital that you serve doctors and trustees, and it's easier to act that way than to deal with community groups and problems.

The easiest way to be a CEO is to be weak. That kind of system looks good on paper—shared responsibility, committees and stuff. But it slows everything down. A fast pace means you must work harder, which is the way you achieve goals. It's easier to work through committees: no single individual can be held accountable; it eliminates risk; it can't be "your" mistake, only "our" mistake. I believe in individuals, not groups. Only individuals have imagination, take risks, make grays into blacks and whites. Doing stuff is all there is. If I wanted the other thing, I wouldn't have chosen such a hard job.

There must be a match between the environment and the individual. Van Buren is different from a sophisticated medical center. A competent person can do either job, but Van Buren is homier. The level of sophistication of M.D.'s and the board is different. The managers here have much more administrative responsibility. We don't spend too much time wandering among the various power groups; we have a more corporate arrangement. This place depends on administrators more than a place in which authority is more diverse, confused, and diluted (as in an academic health center, where the university president is involved and the department chairmen have independent powers).

You can only know how good you are after a while, when you look back and see what happened. I believe that even after the first year things appeared better, from improved emergency care in an underserved area to improved institutional morale and a sense that we could do better, we wouldn't be losers anymore. You can look at the record. After 19 years you can see more clearly than you can after 2 or 3 years. Is the institution's ability to serve stronger than it was?

I can't think of any barriers to managing effectively here, other than insufficient funds to do what conscience tells you to do. If you're poor enough, this can be bad too. I don't see barriers at the moment. That could change overnight—the board of trustees could lose confidence in me and feel a need to monitor microbehavior, so I would spend all my time on that. The medical staff could change things too, if they chose to be truly nonsupportive instead of raising questions, blustering a bit. Insensitivity to the community would cause me problems.

The barrier is being so busy defending yourself against what's going on that you have no imagination to do the things you ought to be doing. Any of those groups could create that barrier. Too much oversight by the board creates too much concern about the politics of relationships. You focus on the relationships, not on the organization or the objectives. That's how it works for administrators too. Being so accountable at the micro level eliminates risk taking: you can't operate on instinct or "let's take a chance." The board stays at a macro level here, so the opportunities are marvelous. Our board is well informed on the environment in which we serve. My board chairman gives me the feeling that I can make a mistake. When I came here, the board was oppressive—no administrator had been at Van Buren for more than 3 or 4 years. The medical staff was decent, and they knew it and were strong.

The whole reason I came here was to seize an opportunity born in disaster—to redefine an institution, to broaden the concept of what an institution could mean to a community. I spent 10 years as the chief operating officer of the hospital nearby and was good at the details of my work. You can't be good imaginatively if you don't understand the work at the micro level. I had strong feelings [about health services] because I had received medical care at the local municipal hospital; that was my family doctor. It's no accident that we have a large federal grant for an underserved community—I understand these problems first-hand. This hospital is a neighborhood center of health and well-being services.

My agenda is to understand neighborhood need and adjust resources to meet it. That is both my short-range and long-range agenda. Services for older people are a dominant feature, and we are developing a strong staff of people who can manage social support—that will continue. So will the health center. Some of our neighbors will choose a different way of buying care, so we must remain open to contractual relationships with HMOs. Some loyal doctors are asking

me, Why negotiate with HMOs and make them stronger? I tell them
the hospital must negotiate if some of our neighborhood people so
choose to buy their health care—they own the institution. Doctors
can refuse to negotiate as private businessmen, but we are a com-
munity-owned institution. In some other hospital, doctors might say
they don't believe in this. The administrator might say it could hurt
the hospital financially if it doesn't negotiate. But no one in the room
would say, We are boycotting some of our neighbors because of the
way they want to buy care. The CEO should be more thoughtful and
force the board to be more thoughtful—the contribution that I make.

We're talking about merger possibilities and acquiring a long-term
care unit as a partner. Also, we are trying to improve the performance
of the diagnostic center and our for-profit company. The most difficult
thing is maintaining everyone's confidence and trust to allow one to
do all these things. It's what one does each and every day that main-
tains these. I'm perceived as a strong administrator, but the line between strong and arrogant is anybody's choice, particularly if you're
on the other side of the fence and don't like what I am doing. I need
enough self-confidence for people to think, If he says it's good, it's a
good thing to be doing.

I don't think my job is changing; nor is my effectiveness. You can
only judge effectiveness in hindsight. On a daily basis, it goes up and
down with regard to controversies—if your basic situation is good.
When you lose confidence and trust, the controversies get more intense and diverse.

What I fear about the merger situation is that the honeymoon is
over in terms of what I've built here—I will have to set up new relationships and redefine the role of the institution. There's nothing in
this but trouble for me, but that's what I get paid for. I have the deal
I want right now, what any administrator might want to have—with
a little less pressure on the money side.

I think that institutional costs are insignificant. What's important
are the costs of health care to the society. I always think in those
terms. When we built the housing complex for independent older
people in 1975, we were going to be more than landlords, although
the rules weren't set up for that. I am the president of the complex.
It allows people to live outside of institutions and contains costs.

Inside, because of our never-ending money problems, we have
no fat built into the budget, and the doctors have never dominated the
budget process. Our cost per day reflects this. This is an advantage
in managed care. Our capital cost of $65 million is very low too. That
was one of the most important things we've done here. All institutions
take their existing institution and add to it little by little. I said that

we should get it all done at once or close it. And the building is holding up well. Our operating cost per day is low, and so will our capital cost be—it is—the neighborhood hospitals have spent more like $100 million.

I influence quality through our procedures for putting the right people in the right spots. The board of trustees appoints clinical directors on the recommendation of the search committee (which is composed of other clinical directors plus the CEO, who is president). I always feel I have an independent responsibility, the heaviest weight of responsibility. If they all voted to appoint an individual I didn't approve of, I would tell the board I didn't agree and I think the board would pause. Knowing that to be the case, the discussions of the search committee are altered. You won't find a search committee here who says, This is a medical matter. The questions would not be on the clinical side. For example, all the applicants for a certain position had the right credentials. I felt one of them lacked substance, and I said so. Then we discussed that we had been an all-Italian institution with Italian chiefs and that maybe in this service another Jewish chief would not be right, politically. The candidate lacked ambition. I struggled with these factors and considered whether I should let this person be hired. My view is that the clinical directors report to me and I influence them like another administrative person. I do not play amateur physician. I get stuck with the differences that develop between them. For another example, we must decide whether to extend a chief's appointment beyond age 65. We recommended against it for one individual.

Mine is a great job, I think. I believe in individuals and not in committees. I believe in getting advice. Other people have information and perspective that you need, but you need people who feel individually responsible and accountable. If the board said, You have too dominant a position, then I would say, If you want me to, I would be glad to take it easier. To have committees dilutes my responsibility and risk—no one can be blamed for things that go wrong. This is why groups are created. If we do that, I will have to work half as hard, it will slow the pace down. When things are sent to committees, nothing happens.

Health is one of the things that make us civilized; it's at the top of everyone's priority list. Good health is all there is. Without it you don't have anything. It's too important to leave to those who make a living out of it. I accept regulation, therefore, by public officials, theoretically elected, who then appoint others to carry out that responsibility. And it shouldn't be left solely to those who buy medical care. I have to live with those regulations, and I deal with them as best as I can. I just accept them. I try to take care of the things I can take care of.

Ted Grover, CEO of Cleveland Hospital

Background

Cleveland Hospital has over 500 beds, more than 2,000 employees, and gross revenues of over $100 million. Its primary missions are service and teaching; it is closely affiliated with a local medical school. Cleveland Hospital is believed to be midrange in organizational complexity relative to the other three organizations, because it has two hospital sites and has a teaching, as well as a service, mission. Its environment is believed to be more turbulent than that of either Washington Medical Center or Van Buren Hospital: Cleveland Hospital faces competition from neighboring hospitals with a similar service mix, its patients and physicians are more widely dispersed geographically, and its financial situation leaves little margin for error with regard to acceptable losses from operations.

Ted Grover is in his mid-forties, has a master's degree in public health, has worked at Cleveland Hospital for more than 15 years, and has been CEO for more than five years. He was interviewed on March 28 and June 24, 1986.

Interview

I have been president since 197-, when I was made executive director and CEO of the Cleveland Hospital. In 198-, when we merged, I became president and CEO of the two merged hospitals. Since the 1970s, the CEO has reported directly to the board. The chairman of the board is responsible for presiding over and coordinating the board and has "general" control over affairs. The president is CEO and has "active" control over affairs. If someone takes exception to something I do, I go back to the board rather than to the chairman. This happened a couple of times—once with regard to a budget reduction when a chairman felt the cuts were too deep. We took the plan to the entire committee for discussion and approval. That takes mutual respect and confidence.

I started here in 1968. I never thought I would be here this long. The reason I've continued to stay is that my position has changed relative to my objectives from one year to the next. The board of trustees is an excellent group, made up of people of very high char-

acter who have earned community and professional recognition in
many areas. They demonstrate extreme competence through personal
achievements. You see a professionalism here which is not seen in
other hospitals with regard to the board and the CEO. They don't
look over my shoulder or have unrealistic expectations so long as
general operating objectives are being met. They are a board of trustees holding the hospital in trust and setting policy, not a board of
managers making operating decisions on a monthly basis.

The hospital required substantial physical change to fulfill its purpose in the local community, given that a nearby municipal hospital
(which we were operating under a contract) would be closing. Our
future as a teaching institution and as an adjunct to the private practice of medicine would have been seriously compromised without the
new facilities. We needed a structure for operation independent of
the municipal sector—as a private hospital with expanded ambulatory
care and emergency service and as an academic and tertiary center.
We developed a strategic plan that year to meet those objectives.

I felt that the hospital also needed a friendlier style and a more
cooperative one with its clinical chairmen and medical staff leadership—there was a possibility of a serious break. There had been
extreme hostility, in some cases, to the previous administrator, and
some issues were not necessary to fight over. The hospital also needed
a more focused business plan to accomplish the refinancing. I wanted
to concentrate on the things we could do together and set aside the
things that weren't important, to look the other way on a few things.
I wanted them to view me as fair and thoughtful, to take the edge off
their hostility.

The previous CEO was loved by the board. They thought he was
brilliant, tough, and a cost-effective manager, although a little abrasive. They wondered if they could get someone else as competent.
They were upset when he resigned. He is a private person, but he
told me he'd been talking with the CEO at a larger medical center
about a new position. He said to me, I think you can do this job and
I'll recommend you, but as you know, it will be a board decision. I
told the board chairman, I'm not interested in an acting position, but
it may be necessary because I want the board to look at other candidates; I am here and I can run the hospital. Some people felt others
were better qualified or that they should be considered—it was good
that I left on vacation then. The executive committee decided that,
given my past performance [as associate director] and history (dealing
with the union, medical liability, financial disaster), I should be appointed. This was what I came back to. It was necessary to separate
some people, and some people resigned. The board expected unin-

terrupted operation and fiscal solvency. They knew I knew the plans to get there and I knew the board. Finances then were very difficult, and I entered into a financial reorganization that very year. I was confident that I would rebuild the facility, which some of the trustees and others didn't think we could do. They knew I held the view that the hospital exists for the public health of the community. To achieve that, it needs a satisfied staff, a medical staff engaged in private practice, and a role as an educational institution for physicians.

Having been the associate director, I found the structure was fundamentally acceptable. It merely required more focus. Relationships with medical staff needed more attention. A critical path for refinancing had to be established. We had a team spirit about what we wanted to do. I had been the chief operating officer. When I came in 1968 to work with the executive director and the president, who was the CEO, the hospital was in terrible shape—the facilities were poor, there were major community pressures, we were trying to run education programs and the municipal hospital without full-time chairmen in all major departments, some of the new chairmen didn't have offices, and nothing had been planned for them. Long-range plans and commitments were made without a business or financial plan. In 1972, a commission was developed by the board to reevaluate the hospital—there was fear of bankruptcy. The CEO resigned. The executive director and I served with the consultants to restructure the medical center. Expenses were reduced in medical programs not required and in management. We restructured purchasing, established a new corporate fiscal officer, and developed a complete new finance division. We organized a computer division; closed unnecessary, trendy ambulatory care programs (such as an outreach family health center, for which there was no money); closed the animal research lab; and closed the open-heart surgery program, as a few examples. We also rewrote the corporate bylaws. A very senior board member who ran a multibillion-dollar corporation with only a dozen committees said to me, I suggest only a few committees—finance, operations, medical affairs, and executive—a joint conference committee if you must. I've added development, insurance, and quality assurance since those days. Then we rewrote some sections of our medical staff bylaws. So I was the author of our reconstruction during a period of extreme change and hostility in many areas.

I have a congenial style. I try to factor respect through reasonableness, intelligence, and patience, build a collegial atmosphere around a work effort and ethic: Let's get behind this and make it work. Rather than taking an autocratic approach, I enjoy seeing people excited about objectives. People respond better when they trust you and aren't afraid of you. It's more like love, where there is a mixture of fear of loss and deep respect. Sometimes, circumstances dictate a more direct and aggressive approach, when you have to tell people things that they don't want to hear. It's my job to do that. I try to exhibit enthusiasm to my staff. If the boss doesn't have enthusiasm and faith in the future, others won't have it. I have a major fear that as good people get older and tire, or weary of their workload, or suffer burnout they will develop a short-timer attitude, which is an earmark of a deteriorating organization. No one can tell me the future is bleak, it's just not true. Young men and women who are joining us today will solve problems that existing staff leave behind and could not deal with. The organization must be focused and moving with confidence and enthusiasm.

We never accomplish everything or our goals aren't great enough. I wasn't able to acquire the 400-bed nursing home across the street, as we were going to do, because of changes in state fiscal policy. We still suffer from town and gown problems with attending staff, despite my best efforts.

I have to satisfy the clear objectives of a corporate mandate "to provide accessible, high-quality human services to all persons, with public health programs and medical education as significant institutional responsibilities." I have to be confident that my performance meets the expectations of trustees, regulators, medical staff, and employees. Their own objectives for the hospital must be satisfied. Most important is that the people whom we serve be satisfied. The organization must be stable enough to manage itself without my constant day-to-day involvement—I haven't achieved that, by the way.

There's a performance appraisal of the CEO and senior staff each year by the executive committee. We talk about the organization and our progress or failure in meeting objectives. We also review executive compensation and benefits. There is a sense of progress. If the board didn't have a sense of progress toward and control over goals they set and understand, they would be dissatisfied. We have a formal, strategic business planning and budget process; however, in the executive committee discussion and review, we look specifically at objectives. For example, our professional staff credentialing process isn't as refined and sophisticated as it ought to be, and progress in community renewal around the hospital has been too slow. These are some of the major issues we talk about and around which we plan specific changes. This review occurs in October or November of each year. At the meeting I talk about the vice-president for finance, the executive directors of the two hospitals, the vice-president for development, the associate administrators at both hospitals, the directors of nursing at both hospitals, the planning director, and the vice-president for medical affairs (I don't discuss the clinical chairmen of the departments). There are 16 people to review in two hours. I submit a report on compensation, with comparative data from other hospitals, and an organizational structure for the year. (There are 12 trustee members of the executive committee.) Last year, salary increases ranged from 0 to 16 percent.

To improve relations with the medical school is one of our objectives. I set out to make myself more visible to the president. I'm cochairman of the medical education committee, and I'm more active in the consortium. Things are much better.

The toughest decisions have to do with terminating people. We're all human, and we recognize the limitations of certain people—in some cases we like them. I'm sad about the problems and trouble I've placed into their lives because of business goals (for example, termination of chairmen or an administrator). A second tough function has to do with program issues—the go or no go—for example, closing the family health center or reconstructing our second small hospital. In the latter case, there are a lot of short-range data and thinking indicating that immediate downsizing is appropriate. There is a big risk of building something that will create a liability; however, we made a commitment to the board, local community, and state, based upon sound data, to continue services there when we merged. I'll keep that promise, because the facts remain the same. I have satisfied myself that there are many basic fiscal, business, and public health reasons to rebuild, and we will move ahead even though many disagree—they don't care to understand the facts.

A major pitfall for a person in this job would be complacency. Everything changes. You've got to be ready to change with the times. This is an anxiety-producing, insecure profession. The board must understand your objectives and find them acceptable.

I want to leave behind a reputation for high-quality management and a structure which supports that—and a replacement with those same kinds of qualities.

An effective manager in this organization has the technical ability and vision to understand the need for and impact of change. Implementation of change requires great human skills as well as commitment and compulsiveness.

The executive committee of the board evaluates me relative to their collective expectations. I evaluate myself relative to stated goals and the reactions of my subordinates and peers to what I've been able to—or not able to—accomplish. I try to live up to my own standards. Sometimes I look in the mirror and ask, Have I fulfilled

all my obligations, professional and personal? Have I studied, put in
the time? Am I sensitive to the needs of other people? I have to look
at how subordinates are doing: are they growing and relating positively and honestly?

Barriers to managing effectively often have to do with personality
and social issues within the structure. You must understand them.
You've got to run over them or adapt to them. When you've been
here as long as I have, you recognize and deal with the need for
change, but you're also bound by longstanding loyalties, which can
be difficult to deal with. Ever since the corporation was developed,
dealing with the two sites without a corporate holding structure and
centralized management has been difficult. Having a depressed local
economy and serving extremely ill, often poor people make for a lack
of operating money and access to capital, our biggest constraints on
program and facility development. We are forced to develop
alternatives.

An extremely intelligent and supportive board provides me with
good advice and support when I need it. For example, we withdrew
recognition from the house staff union. We knew it would be difficult.
When we withdrew, the union went all out to force us to change—by
intimidation of the residents, threats, strike, picketing of board members, and political pressure. Board members stayed with us. The same
situation occurred at another hospital in our area, and its board reversed management.

The community being as depressed as it is has provided this hospital with an opportunity to respond through the development of important services that regulators understand are needed. This has made
our arguments for support compelling. Meeting basic needs develops
so much support that you can do more with less and often develop
support in unique ways.

I'm effective and take great pride in what I do. This comes from
my proven ability to accomplish objectives. If I were a little more
hard-hearted, I might be more effective in human relations issues.
When people have problems, I try to help them, so long as they work
at a self-help program. Sometimes it's not worth the effort from an
organizational point of view.

I learned to be an effective manager through very good formal
education and, most important, by working with effective administrators—my role models. I worked with people who conducted themselves professionally and were committed, compassionate people. Like
my board, they gave me an opportunity and believed in me. To this
day, I wouldn't want to let them down—they expect me to do well.
I saw the work ethic of good administrators and saw that things could

be accomplished through enough work and energy. It may all go back to the things we believe in and the way we were trained.

My agenda for the short run is to continue! To create a system offering me challenges and rewards. I've turned down other opportunities as recently as last week. Other jobs aren't much different from what I'm dealing with here, but I know what I'm dealing with here and what I control. I want to be near my family. My long-term goals are:

—To prepare the hospital for the long term. I will foster the best qualities in the basics: sound financial planning; stability; analysis of program design and implementation to insure market viability (because the programs serve and meet real needs); and a state-of-the-art quality assurance program. These goals are achievable through positive relationships with community groups, business groups, insurance companies, and regulators, who will continue to play an important economic and programmatic role.

—To improve and clarify our relationship with the medical staff and the medical school. This will continue to be very important and ever changing.

For the longer term, I intend to continue working toward the development of a regional health system of some sort. It's unfortunate we couldn't pull it off at this time in our area—we are all too big and independent—so we must work out other forms of linkages.

My job is changing to become more policy-oriented. I spend more time outside the hospital on quality of care, malpractice, and reimbursement methodology. That produces problems back in the hospital and puts a lot of strain on me personally.

I think I do the job better now than a few years ago, and I do it differently. As demands change, I'm required to examine how I can best serve the hospital. For example, leading the technical and advisory functions related to the state malpractice bill and insurance rates are extremely important. I've served as chairman of a statewide committee and as chairman of a cooperative insurance company. It's different from anything I've done before. It gives me satisfaction to see major changes in law and insurance come about as a result of my efforts. One decision in the captive insurance company can result in a major change in the bottom line of the hospital. That's why I do it.

How do I view operating costs? They are determined in large part by societal expectations and regulations. There are unavoidable levels of expense related to capital and trained staff (often represented by organized labor), with standards mandated by various agencies in both areas. The administrator has little control over the resultant unit price. We attempt to control costs by sharing and regionalization, but we're quite large by ourselves and rank high among the multisystems in the country. Expense reduction is the result of constant management attention to unnecessary programs and staff caused by changes— you may no longer require certain things. Expense audit is an ongoing process. We bring in others to look at it—consultants and visitors— there are always things you can do to reduce costs. From what we have seen, as a teaching institution, the array of services is appropriate to our area. We haven't done as much in primary care, but I don't think that would have reduced costs. The future is another story, with managed care programs mandating less utilization; however, it's a short-term method of reducing expense per patient illness. It will not cap or reduce total expense levels over time because of the basic fiscal requirements of quality care, public expectations, and new technology.

You can never do enough to insure high quality. It requires constant attention. We've put in place a medical structure—both in terms of concurrent review and retrospective quality assurance monitoring—that insures regular feedback to management and the board. Other critical indicators are patient satisfaction and complaints, which we monitor regularly; medical staff conduct, a key focus in liability problems; and individual and systematic annual review and credentialing, now interrelated processes. We haven't done all we ought to, as a result of the history of our profession. We have dealt professionally with people who have made errors by retraining. During the past few years, I've been requested to use a more punitive system required by regulations. These regulations require a whole new relationship between management and the board. Again my job is changing. My challenge and opportunities are before me.

Sam Woodrow, CEO of Wilson HMO

Background

Wilson is a prepaid group practice plan, or group model health maintenance organization (HMO). It contracts with nine affiliated medical groups to provide care to Wilson members. The Wilson system has over 4,500 employees, with gross revenues of over $700 million. The HMO has over 900,000 members. Wilson HMO's organizational complexity is believed to be high, relative to the other three organizations studied. Unlike the hospitals, Wilson HMO combines financing and delivery of health care. In addition, Wilson interacts with the nine independent medical groups, has several subsidiaries, and has many sites and facilities distributed over a wide geographic area. The environment Wilson operates in is turbulent because a number of well-financed new competitors are entering Wilson's service area.

Sam Woodrow is in his mid-fifties, has a master's degree in public health, and has worked in his present position for more than five years. Previously, he was CEO of another large HMO for more than five years. He was interviewed on December 23, 1985, and July 7, 1986.

Interview

I was elected president of Wilson HMO in May and took the job on a full-time basis in August 1978. At the time, I was very much aware that Wilson had flaws in its structure from the standpoint of a traditional group practice HMO. I had a charge to strengthen the plan and to position it for the future. My first goal was to assess the organization's strengths and weaknesses and to determine the course and shape of any change that was to come.

I had many discussions with ex-Wilson management as well as with medical group and board leadership while I was considering the position. From these discussions it became clear that Wilson had several strengths as well as areas where organization and structure could be improved upon. The strengths were that Wilson had a sizable membership, an established delivery system, a well-known name, and a product, medical care, which should be in increasing demand, given Wilson's favorable premium structure.

However, Wilson did have some significant weaknesses. There were too many participating medical groups that had to engage in significant fee-for-service activity in order to survive and who were, because of their small size, unable to take advantage of economies of scale.

Because the groups had to rely too heavily on fee-for-service patients, there were inherent conflicts in service to plan and nonplan patients. Although the medical groups were performing favorably in terms of hospital utilization, Wilson's failure to underwrite hospital benefits (as of 1978 Wilson only underwrote medical benefits) meant that the savings generated by lower hospital utilization could not be returned for the benefit of the system and its members. This contributed significantly to the plan's undercapitalization, which in turn inhibited the plan and the groups from maintaining first-rate, modern medical facilities and environments. This latter problem was compounded by the fact that Wilson's providers were financially responsible for their facilities, which resulted in unevenness in facility design, location, upkeep, and maintenance.

Membership at this time was limited to a small number of accounts, with the result that membership was stagnating. No growth means slow deterioration; the population ages and needs more services, and the costs of care increase dramatically, resulting in increased premiums that could price the plan out of the marketplace.

In assessing the plan's strengths and weaknesses, I became convinced that Wilson did have a viable product but that it had to become a fully developed prepaid group practice plan in order to succeed. This meant reorganizing the plan in several ways: we had to place control for growth and development in the hands of Wilson; we had to recapture our hospital savings; we needed to convert our medical groups into fewer, larger, more efficient entities which were fully committed to Wilson patients. Finally, if the plan was to succeed and to continue to enjoy its favorable premium, we had to reach out to new markets.

The first step in the process was for Wilson to become an HMO. We did this by becoming state-certified in 1979. This gave us the legal right to underwrite hospital benefits and a mandate to market to new groups. We had to bring our membership under full HMO coverage underwritten by Wilson. To do this we adopted a twofold strategy: all new groups (and we now have added over 1,700 groups in the commercial sector) were to be offered only HMO coverage, while all significant existing accounts would be encouraged to convert to HMO benefits. This strategy proved successful. We now have over 2,000 accounts, all of our major longstanding accounts have converted to HMO coverage, and fully 90 percent of Wilson's account membership is in our HMO plan. By capturing hospital savings, and by raising premiums which had been level for years, we began to generate the capital that made it possible to begin to restructure the program.

For example, Wilson was in a position to provide medical groups with a realistic capitation payment. This facilitated the formation of fewer, more effective medical groups as it became clear to the groups that full-time Wilson practice was economically feasible. Furthermore, we were now in a position to relieve the groups from the financial burden of having to maintain and equip the medical centers within which they practiced. We now have nine regionalized medical groups whose physicians practice on a full-time basis on behalf of Wilson patients. Moreover, the responsibility for developing and maintaining the Wilson system has now been centralized to Wilson, thus enhancing evenness in facilities, equipment, service, and expansion.

By such regionalization, we were able to get an even better handle on hospital utilization than we had previously. With the plan now fully at risk for hospitalization, we were able to provide physicians with reasonable incentives to improve hospital performance. Further, with nine regionalized groups, we were able to centralize our hospitalization in far fewer hospitals, thus enhancing our leverage with hospitals and enabling us to monitor more closely what was going on.

Wilson today is a fully developed, prepaid group practice plan. The strategy appears to have been sound. Our product is still a viable and an attractive one; moreover, the plan is now in as strong a position as it has ever been. We now have our largest membership ever; an account base of over 2,000 covering all sectors of the local economy; a strong delivery system that, although not yet ideal (one medical group would be ideal), is now well managed; and physicians who are more committed to Wilson and the Wilson system. We can still improve, but we now have a structure in place that will facilitate rather than inhibit further progress. Given the onset of the competition now facing us, we couldn't have chosen a better time to put our house in order.

A positive result of our reorganization is that we are now perceived as a dynamic organization that is here to stay. This has enabled us to attract and retain competent managers who in turn add to the esprit de corps of the organization.

When I met with the board search committee initially, I told them what I believed had to be done. Part of the reason they hired me was that they agreed with me on direction and felt I knew how to do it. They said that they wanted a strong leader committed to improving the system, but they were unsure of priorities and implementation. What impressed them was that I had a strong sense of the direction in which I wanted the plan to go. I was committed to prepaid group practice, and I told them that I thought changes had to be made in the structure of the organization. We discussed these issues for a long time. The board was not unmindful that with change there would be some turmoil and that we would be taking considerable risk.

The board and our medical groups were committed to the changes in concept. However, there is quite a difference between conceptualizing a strategy for change and actually implementing it. Merging 26 medical groups into 9 presented real problems to those medical directors affected by the mergers. The board was asked to approve significant capital expenditures which formerly were minimal. Our initial commitments called for $75 million in financing. This was a debt burden of a magnitude Wilson had never before faced. Given the amount of risk involved in accepting underwriting responsibilities for hospitalization for hundreds of thousands of members, the board had every reason to be anxious. This was risk new to the plan which involved an area of expenditure the plan did not have direct control over, and it was occurring at a time when the organization of the groups was in flux. If things had gone wrong, Wilson would have been severely damaged, given the dimensions of the risks we took. Making the changes and assessing the risks took considerable courage on the part of the board and the medical leadership. It showed a lot of confidence in me at an early point in my tenure at Wilson. I think this was in large part a measure of how deep the commitment was to seeing Wilson's program improved, as well as recognition on their part that no change had ceased to be a viable option.

In instituting all these changes, we were converting what had been a status-quo operation into an organization that was to become change-oriented. Overcoming years of acceptance of the status quo was not easy, regardless of the depth of the commitment conceptually to re-organization. Because of the impact of change on our medical groups and the importance of the medical groups to our strategy, I had to win their active support.

Previous executives who had wanted to institute similar change but who had not paid sufficient attention to winning medical group support had lost their jobs. Medical leadership had to be persuaded that change was in their best interest and in the best interest of the organization. If we were going to ask the medical groups to become more interdependent with Wilson, we had to convince them that Wilson could grow, that it could remunerate the groups fairly, and that restructuring would lead to a stronger organization and increased market share.

We had to demonstrate to the groups that we could back up our statements. Increased capitation payments to the groups began to win their confidence. The offer to buy their facilities and equipment and to upgrade them had to be handled by acceptable financing which was reasonably guaranteed. We had to overcome a lot of skepticism at first, which made negotiating the first merger arduous for both sides. However, when the remaining groups saw that Wilson was serious about its intentions and that the commitments were real, the process accelerated.

Our other key constituencies also had to be convinced. We had to assure our organized consumers that service and access would not be diminished as a consequence of greater medical group size. We also needed to show the board some fairly immediate results. We had convinced the board that the financial risk they were taking was a sensible one that could be partially financed by more growth. We had to build a marketing department. (This had been limited.) I had to convince them that Wilson HMO was salable in commercial markets. I brought new staff in, trained them, brought in a new marketing director. We had a few successes, and this enhanced our credibility. We had to convince existing accounts to convert to Wilson HMO. This was difficult when what they had wasn't unacceptable. My argument was that it was premium-efficient and would enable us to control costs more effectively and to enhance our service.

This was a very trying time. We had a lot of new initiatives going, all of which involved risk. They were interdependent. If we had fallen down in one area, it could have damaged significantly our credibility with all our key constituencies. It could have halted all the significant change we were trying to implement.

With a combination of luck and skill we were able to pull it off. Fortunately, I had some things going for me that my predecessor did not: the time was right, the organization was ready for change conceptually, and there was an acceptance of the fact that the organization could not retain the status quo and remain viable. Further, I had extensive experience in the HMO field and was sensitive to the legitimate concerns and needs of the plan's physicians. My skills and experience as a negotiator stood me in good stead in the Wilson environment. I was prepared to avoid brinkmanship to accomplish our goals: if complete reorganization was not feasible immediately, significant movement in the right direction was satisfactory. These negotiating skills might not have been as significant in other environments, but in a constituency-based organization such as Wilson, where give-and-take and flexibility are needed, they proved to be invaluable.

We have made a lot of progress. Our financial performance has been excellent. Physicians are now committed to Wilson and to its success. We have first-rate facilities and modern medical equipment. We've improved amenities. Taken together, we have enhanced the image of Wilson, not only in our own eyes, but in the eyes of our members. Having tasted success, our organization is more aggressive. We are now ready to take on the competition, whereas formerly we might have been more timid. We believe we have a more solid organization, and we project that belief. We can see the results in the way our various publics react to us. I am particularly proud of this last accomplishment—to see how regulators, business leaders, the media, and the provider community view us. It's hard to measure the effect of this on productivity, but I firmly believe it has made a positive impact. People pull harder for an enterprise they feel proud to be affiliated with.

There is still room for improvement in our program. We do not have the kind of efficiency that could be obtained with one medical group. We need to integrate medical services better, have less competition among groups in recruitment of physicians, and share special services more appropriately. There are still some inequities in services and caring in our nine regions. (They are all acceptable, but some areas need further improvement. If we had only one large medical group, I believe this would get us closer to our standard.)

I would like to achieve more in terms of enhancing our image. Wilson is affiliated with some of the finest hospitals in the city. We have a cadre of highly qualified physicians. We have not publicized this adequately. We have not done enough to overcome negative views of Wilson that have been held for many years but are not based on the reality of today. We could have been more sophisticated in our marketing efforts and could have done a better job of tying our facilities planning and development efforts to strategic markets. I recognize in saying this that sometimes my expectations are too high. We had a very small executive team at the beginning of my tenure, and we had to set priorities—and we did. Given what was reasonably doable and the amount of resources that were available, the decisions we made were probably the right ones.

At Wilson, the CEO cannot be completely removed from day-to-day operations. This is and will always be a grass-roots organization. That is one of the strengths of Wilson and can be a source of positive reinforcement, but it can also lead to frustrations. At times, I would like the kind of environment that allows the CEO to devote more of his or her time to the key strategic issues. In a constituency-oriented organization such as Wilson, however, the CEO can never be fully removed from service issues and certain operational matters. A fact of life at Wilson for any CEO is that you will have to involve yourself in hands-on management if you are to succeed. I want to work toward reducing my day-to-day involvement in operations, but I have no illusions that this can be fully accomplished in the Wilson environment. I'm involved in development programs of centers, meetings with consumers, reviews of market strategies, handling of high-level complaints. I'm meeting constantly with senior staff on operational issues, when I'd like to hold them fully accountable for their resolution. I have now a much stronger management team than ever before at Wilson, and they are tackling a larger share of the operational problems than before.

One of the toughest decisions I faced occurred shortly after I arrived. My credibility had not yet been really tested. I was faced with two small medical groups whose care did not meet Wilson standards. I had to confront the possibility that if I took action against these two groups, the other groups would perceive me as being antiphysician at the very time when their cooperation was most needed. If I took no action, my credibility as an implementer of change would be damaged; moreover, it could have been viewed as a willingness on my part to duck the tough issues, something I could ill afford at a time when I was encouraging the board and medical leadership to take considerable risks at my urging. I decided that our program for change would not succeed unless action was taken, and accordingly we notified the two groups of our intention to cancel their contracts unless they merged with other medical groups. In retrospect, this was the right decision, but at the time I was making it, this was a close call.

Going at risk for hospitalization was another tough decision. We are talking here about hundreds of thousands of subscribers. If we had blown our projections and could not handle the risk we had taken, the harm to the organization would have been severe, maybe irreparable. Similarly, the decisions to acquire 55 medical facilities and their related equipment involved great risk. If the additional revenues we were relying upon from increased enrollment, increases in revenue, and hospital savings did not materialize, we would not have been able to honor our commitments. Finally, the conversion of our longstanding accounts to HMO coverage carried great risk. The hospital savings we were counting on would not have materialized if we had experienced heavy losses in membership and could not make up the shortfall with new enrollments. Our marketing program was just getting off the ground, and we had no experiential basis for judging the potential losses in the conversion process. We were fortunate. As it turned out, the risk was well worth taking. We experienced minimal loss in our converting groups and more than made up for the losses with solid growth in new accounts.

Wilson is a complex organization with a complicated history. It is very much an organization by and of its constituent publics. A CEO must understand these nuances to be an effective leader. There will always be give-and-take at Wilson. Our environment is not totally ours to control. We are an important part of the service component of the city and are influenced by this. We also have a social commitment which must be honored—the bottom line cannot be the exclusive rationale in decision making. Accordingly, a CEO at Wilson should never be wedded to corporate ideology. You will be seriously hampered if you come in with specific goals and objectives but lack the management skills to adjust to new situations and new approaches and modifications. Power is fragmented in the Wilson environment; therefore, political skills are necessary to win support for objectives. A traditional business executive would have difficulty, because many of our initial decisions go beyond bottom-line considerations. One example is Wilson's commitment to serving all populations. We will place facilities in markets that competitors would reject as financially undesirable.

Conversely, no CEO can ignore the bottom line without imperiling the company. These competing pressures call for flexibility in the CEO. At Wilson, as at any other organization, you need sound business skills in order to make intelligent business decisions, but at Wilson the demands are much greater than in most business organizations. This is a reasonable compromise for Wilson and an essential component for effective leadership. On the other hand, you cannot compromise on the basics. Flexibility can too often become an excuse for doing nothing.

The CEO needs to balance several, at times competing, priorities in the Wilson environment. It is necessary to take into consideration that our various constituents—the board, organized labor, our medical groups, and major accounts such as the city—may have differing interests on any given issue. I must seek consensus to move forward on major issues, and it often needs to be broad consensus. Moreover, the needs of our constituents must constantly be balanced with Wilson's needs in order to succeed in a highly competitive environment. This calls for strong political and negotiating skills. This also requires the CEO to be out front on issues—to be the consensus builder and not just sit back and wait for it to happen.

An activist CEO is compatible with the Wilson board, if you have the board's confidence. The board will support your plan if it is well thought out and articulated, and the board will give the CEO considerable leeway. This gives the CEO ample room in which to develop new programs. If management fails, however, it will be management's fault; the board will not share in the blame. This degree of confidence in the CEO and his or her decisions is essential at Wilson. When confidence is gone, your effectiveness is too, and you should be prepared to leave.

The Wilson board is a pragmatic board, interested primarily in results. For a strong CEO, this is an ideal situation. For a CEO who looks for reassurance from the board and needs that reassurance in order to act or to validate actions taken, the Wilson environment will be an uncomfortable one.

Evaluation of my performance occurs at two levels. On an ongoing basis, I will know very quickly if the board has lost confidence in me. Conversely, if the board continues to support my proposals as they have, this becomes in essence my review. I do, however, have an annual review with the chairman of the board. This tends to be very results-oriented. I am evaluated on the leadership I have provided. This is a positive experience because it is objective.

It has been difficult to get truly critical feedback from my staff, although the staff is getting stronger in this respect. However, I am the senior corporate officer, and this does put some obvious restraints on the communication process. This phenomenon is not unique to Wilson, and I would have to question any CEO who says that his or her staff is completely free to criticize and therefore constitutes an adequate evaluative body. Some of the staff will be frank with me at times, but even then I have to account for the fact that they may not be fully aware of the decision-making process I had to go through.

I do feel quite strongly that my staff respects me and my judgment. They believe that I have a sense of where I am going and that I know what I am doing.

I believe that I have been a positive leader at Wilson, even if at times I can still be my own worst critic. I do not agonize over decisions the way I used to, particularly when I review our decisions retrospectively. I have learned and am still learning that decisions cannot always be made as perfectly as I might have desired, that if the results we were looking for were in fact achieved, that perfection isn't always necessary to succeed. This is not to say that I have lowered my standards. Rather, I have become more realistic in my expectations of myself and my staff and the complex nature of Wilson.

There were barriers to managing effectively at Wilson and to achieving high standards of performance when I first arrived here. We have overcome many of them, and I think this is another positive aspect of my leadership. The organization had been somewhat stagnant before I arrived, and this had affected the attitudes of Wilson's management. The managers did not want to pursue change and found change threatening. There was a fear of being held accountable which reinforced a bureaucratic mind-set. I had to instill a degree of accountability in the staff and demonstrate that risk taking would be OK. Some rose to the challenge, and others simply left.

We also had to overcome the status quo with regard to the medical groups. We had to come up with economic and psychological incentives to win their support for change. We had to change images of the system and of ourselves that had us believing Wilson was doomed to be weak or mediocre and that this was OK. There was an attitude of, Why rock the boat? Wilson had been doing the same thing for 35 years and it was still here, so why change? There was also skepticism. Who were these new people who felt it so important to have new attitudes, new ideas, and new programs?

Remember, Wilson had been through some very tough periods and had survived. New approaches and "sophisticated" proposals were not treated with awe in the Wilson environment—after all, many new ideas (and their proponents) had come and gone, leaving no discernible impact. There was also concern over my background. Did my experience with other organizations and other structures imply that my coming to Wilson meant change was coming as well?

There were, of course, opportunities to manage effectively. A strong component of the board and of the medical group leadership genuinely welcomed change. But there was some fallout also. The authority I was given, when its impact was felt, was frightening to some. They had wanted a strong leader, but not all of them were expecting so much to happen so quickly. The board was endorsing risk taking on a scale totally new to it in the Wilson environment. Many of our medical directors had not fully thought out the implications for themselves of merging our medical groups. A number of senior Wilson staff had to accept new performance standards and accountability if they wished to stay. People were given real deadlines and quantifiable goals, and they were put on notice that performance would be evaluated. The open-door familiarity of my predecessor was changed immediately, to be replaced by more formal reporting relationships and reporting systems. By moving quickly, I was perhaps too far in front of those for whom gradual change was easier to handle, but I had no choice. If I did not move quickly, opportunity for change would have disappeared.

The organization needs another restructuring and will be ready for it before too long. My direct managerial role must be more limited—too many people report to me; there are too many entities for me to play a direct operational role in all of them. I must be more of a new program developer and policy implementer, and less of a supervisor of operations management at the subsidiary level. It will take two or three years, but the end result will be positive and a less frantic environment for me.

I am hopeful that a more structured relationship between the policy-setting arm of Wilson and its operating entities will allow for appropriate delegations of authority. But structure can only go so far. I must have confidence in the people I am delegating authority to, and the number of people I feel that confident about is limited. Experience, unfortunately, supports a cautious approach. At my previous job there were no more than three or four people I felt comfortable delegating broad responsibility to, and, given the size and diversity of this organization, I need to reach the point where I can have strong confidence in more people. Until that happens, I'll always be spread too thin.

What I've learned is that you can't be a textbook manager. Textbooks set some ideals. You can't be as consistent as you would like to be. The rational manager is nonexistent, relative to the amount of time you spend putting out fires. I learned how to be a leader in the trade union movement. When you win an election and inspire confidence in five to ten thousand blue-collar workers, the leadership principle is similar: they look up to you and follow you. There, leadership was instinctive, it could not be learned in an academic sense. Develop confidence and perform consistently—win grievances, negotiate, reach settlements without losing your followers. It was a huge leap to my next job. I mastered it because I was thrown into it. I learned most effectively by listening.

Brilliant and experienced managers were available to me through our program's close affiliations with a large academic center. Here, I am much more the teacher and lead by example. There, I listened to many conceptualizers who were available to me and absorbed from them. Since I had developed leadership skills, I was in a unique position. I could translate their intellect into actual programs.

My agenda is to mold an organization that can compete as effectively in the future as it does today. That requires continued upgrading of the management and of our service programs (facilities, amenities, systems), a more aggressive posture in the public eye (promoting our positive image, quality, affiliations, facilities, programs, and caring nature), developing compatible new products, and expanding our service area into new markets. If you don't grow, you stagnate. Wilson's own history is proof of this.

We are on a clear path to these objectives. We have a more aggressive market posture. We already have programs in place revitalizing facilities and equipment. We are identifying new service areas. We continue to be positive opportunists and remain open to new things. And we still keep our eye on the bottom line.

We are developing a holding company. I will be CEO of the holding company as well as CEO of Wilson. The holding company is an appropriate vehicle for searching out new ventures. We need one or two more for the near future.

The pressures of overseeing a multistate health system are forcing changes in my present method of operations. The holding company will give me the opportunity to do that. It will force me to concentrate more fully on systemwide issues and new ventures.

In general, our financial position is one of the areas I'm more satisfied with. The model we have is the right one—physicians at financial risk for other than hospital costs. We compare well to systems with which we compete. We probably can do better on the hospital side. We use some expensive hospitals. We might be able to reduce hospitalization further, but there isn't a lot of fat there. When we have more depth in our management, perhaps we could take a fresh look at the resources needed to run our operation. We could be more innovative and more skillful in our use of resources. We could put in some young, bright M.B.A.'s and mix them with experienced staff. You get a dynamic out of this approach, new ways of thinking. I don't think we would have a major impact on productivity with this approach. Our premiums show we are cost-effective. But every little bit helps, particularly in an increasingly competitive market.

On influencing the quality of service, we are undertaking several approaches. We are enhancing the amenities of our facilities, including upgrading the physical plans, interior design, equipment, and support systems. This is part of making the entire organization marketing-conscious. If you want people to have a positive image of themselves and their product, then you must give them adequate tools to work with. We are also working with the leadership attitude in all of our staff, including physicians. This involves a better understanding of the importance of member satisfaction to the success of our product.

Quality of care depends largely on the quality of physicians you recruit and retain. Given our credentialing process, and it's one of the more rigorous I am aware of, the technically deficient physician is usually identified quickly. Moreover, given the attractiveness of a career opportunity at Wilson and the oversupply of physicians in general, we find that we are now able to recruit, in most specialties, some of the best young physicians available today. But credentials only go so far. Accordingly, new physicians are monitored closely by the groups during their first two years before tenure in the system is extended. If the physician is found wanting, he or she will be asked to leave, and this has happened. Even after tenure is granted, there is ongoing monitoring, through our quality assurance programs and medical audits and informally on a day-to-day basis.

There is still some reluctance among the physicians to discipline their peers, but ours is as strong a peer review system as you will find. We, and by this I mean the plan in concert with the physician leadership, are far more aggressive in this area than we used to be. Our performance is good and getting better, something I am particularly proud of given the sensitivity of the issue and the courage forceful action takes.

5.

Interviews with Associates of CEOs

Several associates of the four CEOs were interviewed about a CEO's work and what makes an effective CEO. For continuity and ease of reading, the interview questions (Appendix B) have not been repeated and the responses have been edited.

Regarding Tim George, CEO of Washington Medical Center

Interview with a Clinical Chief

I've been here ten years. I deal with Tim George on all hospital problems, from top to bottom. For example, we have a large burn center. He put up the additional costs as an investment to see if it would work. It's worked spectacularly well. There wasn't one in the city. We've lowered the mortality rate. We're seeing the best survival figures and doing more research. This is one of three research centers funded by NIH. If Tim George hadn't wanted to build it, we couldn't have gone ahead. He helped us with community board approvals and so forth.

Tim is an M.D., and a lot of hospital directors are not. Institutions like this function better with someone of his background in the post. Board members don't understand this. Economically, we would never have built the burn center. A non-M.D. would have no feel for it at all. The burn center does fine economically now; it loses a little money, but the community service is phenomenal.

Long-range planning has been well thought out, financed, grants offered to do it. Managed care is being looked at as hard as it can be analyzed. He's always in on the appointment of professional people. The dean and the director are always involved in this. They need to work together—staff have joint appointments, in the hospital and the medical school. In some hospitals there are major rifts between the hospital and the academic side, but not here.

I see Tim at least three or four times a week apart from formal meetings. I see him on an individual basis about various things—personnel, operating rooms, whatever.

Like most of us, Tim has a staff with responsibilities broken down; he meets with them to describe who's going to implement what and how. He goes to a lot of meetings and does a lot himself.

Right now, he's trying to maintain a good operation in the face of regulation and managed care. In most states, you don't even know who the state health commissioner is. Tim spends a lot of time on regulation and managed care.

His power comes through the board and meeting with its committees. Most of his power comes through the position.

Tim is a good manager. A couple of his people needed to be changed—one was changed, one will be changed. People say that this should have been done earlier. Most of his people have been OK. He's better than most hospital directors—his whole view of medicine is better. He's had honors reflecting that from leadership associations; he's held offices in them. His are not knee-jerk reactions to regulations but careful, considered decisions on the issues. In some places, you have center directors [chiefs] directing grants who aren't responsible to organizational objectives and patients. Tim works well within the system without disrupting their efforts. This is a result of his own efforts and of working with the people concerned. This is a major problem in some places: the policy under which center directors work is important. One center was spun off as an independent research group; this was done on an outside contract basis. It's been done both ways, depending on the thrust of a center, which I think is good.

He is a very stable, amiable, thoughtful fellow, well respected here, regionally, and nationally.

I would rate Tim's performance as excellent. He keeps a major operation going harmoniously. Complaints about him are mostly minor, compared to those about CEOs in institutions of this size elsewhere. Clashes between the voluntary physicians and the hospital occur elsewhere almost to the exclusion of the institution's needs. Practitioner complaints are related to practice. Some hospitals are not responsive to academic needs. Tim won't do things if the monies aren't there, unlike other places.

His techniques haven't changed over time. He's changed in response to changes in the system—the regulators, the strengths and weaknesses of the staff—what he's had to do to keep a big operation going. With managed care, we shall have to make changes. Hopefully, the way it's done, as with other changes, will be so as to get the best possible out of it. If you don't watch economics, they'll be dictating to you how to run the hospital.

Costs were watched all across the board, in personnel, equipment, supplies, and salaries. There is continuing surveillance; everyone's aware of cost-benefit ratios. When costs change, they react to it and do something about it.

Tim influences quality through selection of personnel. He's responsive to new technology as well. He sees every candidate for every major position, helps determine whether they get hired.

In most hospitals outside the Northeast, hospital directors are not M.D.'s. It's almost impossible to translate the patient care implications of cost-effectiveness or quality to them. I've dealt with them. Non-M.D.'s are at a big disadvantage not knowing medicine; they're at the mercy of the people giving them medical input, as far as knowing what the priorities should be. This doesn't result in as good an operation.

The hospital administrator's job depends on the whims of the practicing staff, and the administrator knows that. This makes for different priorities.

At a hospital I know, last week was the first time the hospital director met with all the chiefs at one time. Administrators maintain power by playing off one chief against another and against the voluntary staff. It takes a good manager to do things openly. The chiefs at those hospitals need a surveillance system to know about deals that will affect them. That's a major thing I appreciate in working here. That kind of politics can be extremely time-consuming.

The dean and director meet twice a week. This is important—it gets rid of a lot of that divide and conquer business. Deans use it as well as hospital directors. Meetings dispel that secret service stuff. There are places where the dean and director don't help each other, don't meet, have their own initiatives, and have collisions.

Unitary management of the medical school would be a disadvantage here: one institution would be favored. No one has both types of expertise. The present system works well.

Interview with a Center Director

I head an institute which is a spinoff from the hospital. Tim George was helpful in setting us up. It was designed so we wouldn't have to go through academic red tape in working with government, business, and other institutions. Dialysis was always controversial. No one wanted it, and we got kicked out of medicine when we set it up. We are a premium transplant center. Five years ago the dean and director spoke to me about new ways of financing our enterprise, to work with industry and share profits. Tim led the fight with the state health department to make us separate. It's worked out better than we dreamed. No one should get more credit than Tim for establishing this. We couldn't have done it without him.

I knew Tim as a medical student. We were members of the same department. I recommended to the dean that Tim be appointed as director of the hospital.

The hospital had a problem with high mortality surrounding heart surgery. I got all the charts on deaths and set up a blue-ribbon committee to review them. One change we made was to bring in internists to monitor surgical patients—attendings who were good 20 years before needed educational programs. There were dramatic drops in mortality afterwards. Tim provided what we needed and helped develop it all. You need to do this [quality assurance] with delicacy, which Tim has more of than I do. Tim is a master at that. In the end, the affiliations program was succeeding so well I got accused of conflict of interest; by filling up the hospital I, according to attendings, hurt quality.

We in this organization are a very heterogeneous group with different agendas. How do you orchestrate those agendas and deal with a medical college that feels it should run the hospital without having the qualifications to do so? How deal with practitioners who use the hospital, have given a lot, but who haven't kept up? How deal with people like me who have big ideas of our own, and how deal with others—when we need space and money? How deal with department heads still not imbued with the modern necessity of working together (for example, having an open-bed policy rather than bed allocations)? How deal with the nursing profession, which has changed dramatically over the last 25 years, wanting to assume the role of M.D.'s when there weren't enough M.D.'s? Now that there are too many M.D.'s, how get rid of the nursing school, which isn't cost-effective any more? How keep the unions out? How deal with regulatory agencies? It's an impossible job.

Tim must deal with his own staff and the board of governors. How balance them all off and pick out the right ones to work with? Someone is always angry at the director, and they may have a case, but they don't see the other side. They may be better off if they don't open their mouths, but they don't realize this. Tim has an equanimity and imperturbability that is ideal for the job.

Tim's done good things for me. He's kept unions out of the hospital. He's kept us financially viable. Although the hospital is 50 years old, most things are state-of-the-art. He's walked the line at the medical school and admirably, with people viciously trying to take his job, withstood their attacks and held things together. His staff is devoted to him, although people criticize them. All past deans would attack the staff for apparently justifiable reasons, but he never attacked back.

I'll call Tim on the phone. I usually don't have formal meetings. I'll drop down and see him. It's never very long—10 to 15 minutes. The dean is concerned about affiliations again, and I talked to the two of them for 30 to 45 minutes. It was the dean's meeting.

Tim gets things done through the system he set up. In the hospital he has a lot of power, which the deans have envied, over his people. He recognizes the limitations of his power. You can get frustrated with him that way. I've gotten angry with him about this but realized subsequently that he couldn't do what I wanted. Or that what I wanted didn't need to be done, with the benefit of hindsight.

What I've learned is that Tim's main interest is doing a job. Some of our objections don't relate to the job he's doing, so they get ignored. At times I've been furious with him. For example, in the affiliations program, I didn't want committees, I wanted authority. They made me associate dean and associate director; I became a member of the executive faculty but not of the medical board. He said it didn't make any difference in getting the job done. He was right. He said he would do it [make me a member of the medical board], and he couldn't do it, and I wasn't succeeding as I wanted to, so I was angry.

There's talk now that Tim is leaving and a search committee will look for a replacement. I haven't talked to him about this. He's still trying to steer a course where the hospital would be separate. We're setting up a lipid center with the hospital, and there's a new world of cancer treatment that we're working on. As an institute, we don't have to go through department heads. For example, at the next board of governors meeting the hospital will vote $2.1 million to establish the lipid control center with us. Tim's role is significant in saying it's important for the hospital. We're getting space too.

As a person, Tim is a man of the utmost integrity and honesty. Tim is equal to anyone I've known in these respects. He's thoroughly devoted to principles of medicine and good medical care. He always considers academic benefits and the good practice of medicine as well as budget. Other hospital directors lack his academic sense.

As a manager, he's been criticized. As I look at it from a distance, I think he's an excellent manager. When I ran the kidney center I used to scream, I need more nurses and staff. When I had to start paying the nurses, I changed my tune. Attendings don't like the way rooms are kept, but it's a 50-year-old building. Other hospitals aren't as clean as they used to be either. Tim takes a broader view than deans of the medical school, who don't fully comprehend the hospital side.

I rate Tim's performance as excellent, although there were times I didn't do that because I felt that I was justified in my criticisms. If someone has a good argument, Tim will always listen. I couldn't get anything from Tim without a detailed plan, including finances. He looked in thoroughly on what was necessary. He was an advocate of our institute, but only after we had done our homework.

Tim has developed a broader perspective over time, and he has learned. Good judgment comes from bad experience. He's experienced what anyone in the hospital field has experienced. The people who were against us are no longer here. He's very loyal to the people who have worked for him. If he's erred, it's been in keeping people longer than he should. He has let incompetent people go, but it's painful for him to do so.

Everyone would say he has tremendous integrity. Some deans would say he's a terrible manager because they wanted to manage the hospital themselves. Board members see the complexities of hospital management when they get into it. As a hospital director, Tim would come out better than most—they are whipping boys. People say he doesn't get along with the state health commissioner, but I think this is not the case.

In forming our institution, Tim steered it through all the regulatory agencies. We had gotten through one of the first committees, which never rejects anything, but it rejected us. He called the commissioner and said we weren't understood, and the meeting was rescheduled. He called in a nice way and was persistent.

I remember his being viciously attacked by a former dean. Tim reacted to that with much more equanimity than I would have—I would have been furious.

Tim has a lot of influence on costs. If he doesn't want it, it doesn't happen. The board waits to see what Tim has to say. They trust his judgment. He's kept the union out. Tim has the most power here, which has burned the deans up. He controls most of the budgets.

Tim's had a great deal of impact on quality. I know this personally. I had all the money I needed to do quality assurance, hundreds of thousands of dollars. I've been out of that for four years. I'm not satisfied with what they're doing now, but they're doing a good job. There are a thousand M.D.'s here. I used to have private sessions on who would be watched and who wouldn't be watched. The administration gave that top priority. How do you deal with poor physicians? Tim would back every scheme we could think of. Tim has been the leader of that.

Over 20 years ago, the professor of medicine attacked the artificial kidney. I said I was through. We got out of the department of medicine. The only person who went to the chairman and said he shouldn't do this was Tim. This was the kind of group that attacked Tim. The deans were jealous of Tim's power, and they didn't recognize it themselves. Hospital budgets dwarfed the college's budget.

Interview with an Administrator

Most issues on which we worked have been finance-related, for example, section 227 problems, which involved staff physicians being paid under Medicare. Also, organizing for programmatic issues on the clinical side—this involved assessments of each department. I represented Tim in comparing his assessments with the dean's assessments. I work with Tim on priorities and strategies. The planning process serves as a blueprint for fund raising. I deal with him on the issues of the day also. At present this includes managed care and capital financing. I represent Tim in Washington when he can't go. I spend a lot of time mediating or getting a problem on the table between the hospital and the college.

This is an academic medical center. You must accept the fact that power rests with the clinical chairmen and nurture that. Some are more powerful than others. Intelligence, personality, and resources determine their power. Medicine and surgery chiefs are powerful. Tim recognizes that. To be truly effective, he must touch base with a lot of people. You can turn the board around faster if you tell them the chiefs are behind you than the other way around.

Secondly, this is a human service business. Dealing with people means you must be able to listen and have the patience to listen. Board members tend to come from a different kind of environment.

Clinical chiefs are not analogous to division presidents in business. There have been more successful palace revolts in academic medical centers than at Citibank.

Tim has consistently demonstrated an ability to convey to everyone that, even in the wildest storm, everything is fine and calm; he projects that. Tim insists on looking at things from a nonpersonal perspective—what is best for everyone else, putting himself last. I don't find this too often in hospital CEOs.

His successes have been mobilizing the place, improving the place financially, and continuing in a crazy period to advance delivery here to the cutting edge—we have the first lithotriptor and MRI. He recruits quality academic leaders. Tim's biggest weakness is his loyalty to people he's recruited; he is uneasy about dealing with their human failings and accepting the fact that people change over time and adjustments have to be made. He tends to wait for a crisis before he deals with it. Tim gives you the performance appraisal forms to fill out on yourself—he finds that process difficult. He has no problem dealing with a medical matter, with the professional quality of care.

Tim recognizes that one has to decide on matters for the short term or long term, and he sees that the long-term impact may be more important. Sometimes that gets him into trouble, because people think he's procrastinating. Managed care is an example. Other hospitals went in for an equity position with Maxicare; now they find they can't deal with other insurance players.

I try to touch base with Tim every morning. He's better then. It's very informal, no set format. To really get Tim to react, it's got to be in writing. We used to spend Friday afternoons together, my being his student; that was very helpful to me. He's wise and a good teacher.

Tim gets things done by first touching base with people who are important in implementation, with people who've had experience on a similar issue. He builds a data base and explores different ways to proceed. He elicits others' ideas to build consensus. This makes implementation easier. He's more concerned with success two years from now than with making the decision now. Tim is here for the long pull.

Tim's more of a committee chairman than an autocrat. He's very programmatic. He's patient and deliberate and tries to avoid surprises and glitches. He has no ego as a manager. It doesn't matter to him whether he gets the credit, so long as the thing gets done.

As a person, he is Mr. Integrity, honor and integrity. He takes the position which is best for the institution.

I would rate his performance A− or B+; no one should get an A. Anyone who can survive here for over 20 years has to be doing something right. He took us through difficult times, and the place is poised to be substantially better when he leaves. He's determined to get renovation approval for inpatient facilities.

For the most part he hasn't really changed. Tim is always a learner, doesn't profess to be an expert, is always open to new ideas. Because of increased demands on his time, he's had to make decisions on how he spends his time; and since the former director of nursing's retirement, he isn't as much in tune on delivery issues. His data base is built from a lot of people. He doesn't have time to walk the floors now. He recognizes that this is a problem and is trying to redress it. Given his druthers, he'd enjoy being chief operating officer more than CEO, I think. He'd rather be a doctor than a shill or a speaker.

Tim's been a proponent of being a leader in introducing new technology (for example, CCUs). This has been very costly. We're not being paid for our lithotriptor; he doesn't think twice about that. He looks at budgets as his own dollars and is tightfisted about routine matters.

He scrutinizes the financials. Tim pushed for a financial tool to review DRGs, to put on one page what he needs to know. He looks at the census every morning. A CEO knows if the census is down to get on the phone and get some patients in the house.

Tim has clinical credentials. I think he's had a big effect on quality. He believes quality begins with the chairman.

Sometimes Tim's assumed that the chairmen are as diligent as he is. He established a patient services representative program. That is his audit process. Every administrator hears from doctors and board members about patient care. This is how he hears from patients and their families. He reads or used to read all letters that come in from patients. He's not as in touch with those things as he used to be, and he would like to get back in touch.

In summary: Tim is often misjudged and misinterpreted as not being very impressive. But he's not trying to be impressive or dominate at any moment. He should be judged on his overall track record, over the long run, or on specific matters.

Among our peers, our length of stay is the lowest and our costs are the lowest. We win popularity polls of independent deans and directors—they told us we had the best array of clinical leadership around the country. We got money to look at this from Mellon, for an eight-person panel of deans and directors from other parts of the country. They interviewed chiefs and looked at their plans. They agreed with Tim's assessments.

When Tim came on board, this medical center was dominated by researchers. Now it has a more balanced array of clinical expertise.

The goal of the place is to be preeminent in all three aspects of mission [patient care, research, and teaching]. There was debate over whether this was possible or whether we were to be no different from anyone else, but what was different was that we could do it. We are devoting attention to getting research straightened away. The second biggest issue is facilities renovation, which we are also trying to address.

Tim gives you a lot of latitude, which gives you confidence. He doesn't like surprises, that's all; so it's important to brief him. He disciplines humanely and constructively, as a good professor does with his students. People are concerned about losing Tim's influence as a stabilizer; who will provide that when he's gone?

Interview with Another Administrator

I work with Tim on issues that will change policy or on implementation of new policy. At the beginning, I didn't have my own credibility, and I didn't know what I was doing. Now I go to him only when policy needs to be made at a higher level; when legal cases have a criminal aspect, liability; when bad press can be important; or when it involves projects Tim's working on.

We're not owned by the university; there are tensions of separate and equal status. There is tension over mission, balancing academic and clinical. Here chiefs are prominent, with enormous egos and agendas which may not be the administration's. There is a good old boy circle; some chairmen are more in than others. There are normal tensions of nurses and doctors (here nurses will challenge doctors on an order); the financial world of this state and its regulatory agencies; patient care, teaching, and research; and all that. The environment's changing. The hospital is trying to be all things to all people—a community hospital, a tertiary care center, and a provider of managed care. It's like a mine field Tim must walk through every day—and decisions to take care of one set of problems may upset the balance on the other side. We have 5,000 employees on different levels, environmental regulations, safety issues. And it's an old physical plant: people's expectations are shocked by our facility.

Tim's done a lot. He's recruited 11 new chairmen. (He's dealt with half-dead wood in some of those positions.) He's worked on the building program, our space problems. He established and has given support for patient services. He does a lot quietly.

I interact with Tim formally. When I need him, I get to see him. Sometimes I stick my head in or set up a specific time, depending on the issues. I'm here early and late, so I can see him then.

He delegates a lot. He relies on one administrator a lot for long-range planning and managed care. He delegates a lot to the COO. Tim asks for a plan and then decides, or he reflects and decides at the medical board meeting.

His agenda now is to get inpatient units renovated at all costs and to get managed care off the ground—probably equal in emphasis. And to make this place survive.

He is enormously respected by the medical staff for his accomplishments and the respect he has from employees. He's the sole reason we're not unionized. He's fair. He is respected by the clinical chairmen and members of the board, but not by all of them. He's survived.

Tim's not reactive. He likes to think things through. He's reflective. He's not demanding enough. There are times when you have to be tough, and I would like him to act earlier than he does. He's fair. He gets as much input as he can. He's not autocratic. When he finally makes a decision, he's thought it through, covered all the bases, and it's a good decision. Getting him to that point is the struggle.

He's Jimmy Stewart, Mr. Smith goes to Washington, a sense of humor, he's fair. He's directed mainly toward his work. He works less than he used to do. He is moral, ethical.

He's changed over the last few years. He's more distracted. The outside environment is the most obnoxious it's ever been. In the last five years, he's been forced to deal with things he hasn't necessarily wanted to deal with. He's not as close to the new board chairman as he was to the old one. Tim's very good.

He matches this place. He knows this place and the players. He gets done what has to be done, sometimes in spite of this place and these players. Some talk of a business type replacing him, but the board doesn't understand that you can't run this hospital like U.S. Steel—Tim's big battle. At U.S. Steel you can make steel sheets of different standard sizes, but no two patients are alike—some don't fit the mold, and the system, within reason, must respond to those patients. Tim realizes this. You can't streamline professionals beyond a certain point either. I'm not sure business people understand that.

Changes—three to four years ago, Tim involved more senior people in the decision-making process, a positive move. He expanded the director's staff meeting. Tim's not a great communicator. He says something in a room, and he assumes everyone has heard it. I don't sit in on the meetings, and I don't know what's going on. At least indirectly, he needs to ensure that the word gets out to department heads. We're going to try to do that this year, have him communicate directly with them (about managed care, for example, to dispel rumors and give out accurate information). Just exposing them to Tim will be an uplift. Those who've been around the hospital a while respect him, they know he's fair, they see him during rounds in the evenings and early in the morning. He's not pretentious or filled with self-importance. He doesn't care about his clothes. He's not hung up on material things. He never pursues his greater glory to the exclusion of the institution and the people in it, unlike others.

As to influencing quality, if something isn't done the way it should be, Tim is willing to speak to a chief to see that the problem is dealt with swiftly. He is swift on clinical issues, the physician in him rises to the occasion. He has little patience with poor medical care. The few times I've seen him angry were on patient care issues. For example, in one department, attendants, house staff, and clinicians did not comply with our new do-not-resuscitate guidelines, putting themselves and the institution at risk. He still had the wounds of an earlier case in which an 87-year-old lady was not resuscitated and the hospital received bad press as a result.

Regarding Larry Martin, CEO of Van Buren Hospital

Interview with the Chairman of the Board

Larry began in June 196-. I became board leader in December of that year. The old board had let go of the previous administrator. The first burden became finding someone. We recognized that Van Buren was having more trouble when other places weren't. We wanted someone with experience in this city. We interviewed. Larry had written expressing his interest; he was an assistant administrator at a respected, well-run hospital nearby which was also church-related. He was the right age, 36, had been there for ten years. He came in for an interview. He came across well. We didn't have to move him from another city. I knew enough to know we needed a good guy. As a board member, you're in a position to take a risk which you might not take with your own money. Take the younger, more aggressive guy—the place was in such disastrous shape, we had to rock boats. To some extent, the place becomes a shadow of the guy you take.

Now I have absolute confidence in Larry. He's careful to make sure I'm not surprised. His record is such and our comfort level is such that what he wants to do, we do. In the beginning we were concerned with how we could build a new Van Buren Hospital. I believed that Larry could run the hospital and that the medical staff would be responsive—they were the only good thing we had. In the late 1960s Larry realized that, if we did the neighborhood thing right, we would survive. Larry didn't dream that up in one day. Another hospital began to move in with a mental health clinic and other things. How we protected ourselves was typical Larry—he got grants, he got our congressman involved, he captured that movement in time and made it pay off for us. We got the attention of the community. We used them, but for their own good; we served community needs.

Most hospital administrators have never done anything else, grew up in the business. It's not an easy business to switch into later in life. Larry knows more about the hospital business than I do, so I decided not to meddle. Obtaining voluntary money was where the equity came from for the hospital. My role was to do what Larry couldn't do—fund raising—the almost $3 million that was raised, with the help of an aggressive development guy. I did close the nursing school and the medical records school before Larry got here. Larry didn't want to close the nursing school. We scrambled in the beginning together. The board was weak. We talked to the city about their giving us a municipal hospital, buying land from the Catholic Church (we bought a piece of land) to find a place for the hospital. The development guy came up with the idea of converting this building for hospital use. We asked the city for the property, and the city gave it to us. The architect said we could convert the building. On the inside issues—medical staff, equipment, allocation of resources—I let Larry take over. He knew the business, and I didn't.

Hospitals have a weird management arrangement. A board is legally responsible. The employees are responsible to on-site management. The medical staff controls the marketing effort: patients go to the hospital their doctor chooses. Doctors control market and expenses. What Larry did early on was to establish himself as a strong figure with the physicians. Obviously he ran a good shop and attracted talented people. It's more difficult to run a hospital than a business because of the medical staff problem. You must understand what your mission is. We always understood that we would be a community institution serving our two local communities. The CEO must be strong enough to stand up to medical staff pressure and have the doctors' respect so they will be helpful. Larry tried to involve the chiefs as comanagers, which was unique at that time, so they would feel an institutional responsibility beyond that for their departments. They must feel loyalty not just to the place, but to running it right. Senior physicians should feel responsible for managing the place. Larry had lunch with them every Tuesday; this was an organized forum in front of their peers. I would say to a chief, Don't talk to me about a problem; you figure out a system that is right. Physicians should make these decisions among themselves (for example, admissions priorities when there are not enough beds). Decisions should be made by those who are knowledgeable.

Larry has taken advantage of the concept of serving the community—politicians and people who live there will love us. Make decisions based *not* on your ego, on what the medical staff wants, or on keeping up with the Joneses. The hospital belongs to the neighborhood. Getting that message across to the board, medical staff, and church has been Larry's greatest accomplishment. The neighborhood needs us to do things. We had paid $1.6 million for the property and couldn't sell it for that, so what should we do with it? What does the neighborhood need that we can find a way to do? How do we get the financing?

Two telephone conversations a week—Larry is telling me what's happening. The first few years, he ran every significant management decision by me. I made myself available to him. The hospital was 12 blocks away from my business. It was an important thing for me. The relationship, a unique one, changed over time as Larry got more confidence.

Larry does things quickly once a decision is made. He thinks through where he's trying to go—he's very thoughtful. Larry knows that he has the support of the board. He can blame things on me. He has a gigantic ego; he is an ambitious man. My job is to stand in the background and channel his energy. He's a little like Ronald Reagan— he's not trying to impress his advisers, but he makes good decisions. He creates an environment of strength and confidence; the hospital looks bigger than it is. He's very bright and articulate. He hasn't stood still. He's developed with the business.

Larry sees the health delivery system changing. Ideally, the four local hospitals should band together; they should be one place. We are making ourselves indispensable to the regulators and to the market. He is not just responding; he is trying to create a setting where we thrive, not merely survive. We think this is done by joining with our neighbors. We want to be so important that the regulators can't underreimburse us out of business. We want to be an indispensable part of the delivery system, continue to be innovative; we want the HMOs and PPOs to have to come through us. Right now our focus is to be bigger so that we can be better and be here tomorrow. There's little conflict and misunderstanding now between Larry and me. The psychic income for me has been tremendous. Larry's salary is an easy negotiation, a combination of what he thinks and what they do at neighboring hospitals.

Larry's source of power is Larry. The board is like a corporate board; M.D.'s are vice-presidents, and Larry is president. One of our chiefs feels that Larry rides roughshod over the medical staff. I don't think so. Someone has to be in charge of the economic consequences of what physicians do. There's going to be a quality factor in the competitive market. Larry and I have talked about that; but the talks are less and less frequent.

Larry is bright. He takes his intellectual skills and makes things happen. He's respected. He knows he has the power. But you have to keep the physicians aboard. He understands what has to be done and uses power effectively to get it done. He's surrounded himself with some pretty talented people, and he's backed them.

He is very ambitious as a person. He has a gigantic ego. There's no room for two stars. I know that Larry is the star. I'm the star in my business. It doesn't bother me.

I rate his performance as really first-class. Results speak for themselves, the innovative programs. For a place of this size, the attitude is good. How do you create that? By answering the question, Why are you here? with, To help your neighbor.

Larry hasn't really changed. He's gotten better, in terms of interpersonal relationships. Being successful because of your track record allows you to do things more easily. He's been a risk taker—in jumping the size of the place, creating the imaging center—where his peers aren't so willing to take risks. He has an entrepreneurial streak.

He's perfectly straight, says what he means, means what he says. This has stood him in good stead. Larry's only defect is occasionally acting like a wise guy when he shouldn't, but he doesn't do that so much any more. He's thought out where he wants to be and how he's going to get there. He has a business plan and a strategy, and he sticks with it.

Larry influences costs probably in staffing, administratively, and in total staffing. There is tight control on capital expenditure. We were slower than we should have been getting a CT scanner and cobalt therapy. His attitude was, Use the service at a neighboring hospital; we're a primary care hospital. He doesn't allow professional staff to satisfy their egos. We don't do things that other people can do better.

Larry influences quality by hurting a bit when things go wrong and letting people see this. People make mistakes under pressure. By talking about it, people on the line understand it's important to top management. Larry sets the tone and the atmosphere. He makes the associate administrator understand it's an important part of her job, makes the job as important as it should be. Quality is an important competitive point.

In Larry, you have a unique personality—the right intellectual equipment, a sense of how you get things done in an organization, style in the use of power and creating an environment. When we compare Van Buren's clinical and educational programs with those of other local hospitals, we look good. Larry understands what it is and sticks to it—the key thing—and it's served us well. He doesn't get diverted with the latest technology. Good managers are born, not made. That creative spark—you can't learn it in school.

Interview with an Administrator

I've worked with Larry for many years. Last June I moved into a new role, which is still evolving, and report directly to Larry. I work closely with him on the company [the for-profit activities], the nursing home, programs for the elderly, merger, HMO development [managed care products from outside vendors], image building, and marketing.

[One needs to understand in this business] the dynamics of the medical staff and the interests of the practicing physician. These are different from the interests of corporate clinical directors, who have a role in the institution but are not representative of the practicing physician. Our guys don't always lead the way they are supposed to. For most of our doctors most of the time, their personal interests are paramount. They want a hassle-free institution so they can do what they want for their patients and bill accordingly, without any institutional responsibility. Medical directors have a responsibility transcending that.

In most hospitals, administrative people get bogged down in detail and think they're working in a crisis institution—and they fret about it. In our hospital, the CEO has been successful because he's worked at a level above that; he sees himself as an executive and a leader. He influences the direction instead of carrying it out. He's got to be something of a visionary, to have good intuition in order to know what's real and not real in the environment, where we should be moving. We're basically a community institution with responsibility for a certain population—to meet their basic health care needs, moving beyond medical care where we can. Health is more than taking care of sickness.

Larry has incredible respect for what's important to doctors, the private practice of medicine. He's never done anything to undermine that. With the health center, we never did anything to impinge on [their practice in] the other local community. Same with the HMO—we wouldn't compete with our M.D.'s in that community. Even now, we're organizing delivery systems in areas where our doctors don't practice. Regarding the IPA, we have to be open to any doctors who want to sign with an HMO, not just to those forming the IPA. There are two camps of private practitioners. We support the IPA but won't work exclusively with those physicians. It's a confrontational issue in some hospitals.

The biggest thing Larry did was the new building, the survival of Van Buren Hospital, which was probably on the hit list in the late 1970s. Based on what we were doing, we shouldn't have survived. It took vision to apply for the OEO grant and to see that the partnership with the city health department could be sold. We had nothing to lose in moving here, but it was crazy. And we did the housing complex for the elderly at the same time with basically no money.

He is supremely confident. When Larry left the other hospital, they gave him a pencil without an eraser. He's confident even when wrong. He's smart enough; he always has an answer.

I interact with him usually on an ad hoc basis. We'll make an appointment if it involves someone from the outside. If someone else is there, I pop in with my agenda at the end. Once you go in, it's hard to get out in less than an hour. When he initiates the contact, it's about a specific issue. I tend to accumulate things before I go in.

Larry makes quick decisions about what actions should be taken and how they should be carried out with a group of people. He will decide what it all means and what should be done. He tells stories. It's like tuning into a soap opera, consistent. If you are familiar with the big picture, it's hard to tell when something really happened, or when was the time yes or no was said.

He gives all of us freedom. He wants us to keep him informed. We can turn to him for help. If things are complicated, we can simplify. He lets go of things easily, but you have to know when to touch base with him. On shifts in direction, he's going to be involved. He'll say, That's something I'm interested in.

We're into the next big thing—creating a health care system in this region. It started with one neighboring hospital, and now it's with another one. It will involve merger, vertical integration, managed care, capitated contracts, and foundation grants.

Larry's winning streak is a source of power. He came in here, to an institution that was bankrupt, confident. He hasn't made any big mistakes. He said that corporate consolidation with the hospital where he used to work was right, and its board committee said consolidation was right, but they weren't willing to do it. He's taken the criticism of that hospital's medical staff toward him and used it to show that no one's in charge there.

Larry is different. He doesn't use meetings and committees. He tends to exert strong authority while giving people a sense of freedom. He deals with people on an individual basis. There's an appearance that the CEO operates autonomously, but he talks about a lot of things. Larry's intuitive. It works in a nice way. He's very complex. He likes people to think he's into feelings, but he's uncomfortable about feelings. People therefore think he's cool and reserved. He's very well organized and compulsively neat.

I rate his performance as absolutely superb. He's an incredible person, very smart, and he has a wonderful way of getting people to do what needs to be done. He is ten steps ahead of most people. At executive committees and board meetings he shows this. He says, That's not the way it is at all; this is what it is. He hasn't changed much.

He influenced costs a long time ago, by establishing our scope of services—we would be a secondary institution. Other secondary institutions wanted at least one service they would be known for. He thought this was empire building and setting the wrong priorities. He wanted us to be a good community hospital.

Our getting that OEO grant, which became our outpatient department, put us ahead of a lot of other hospitals, which were drained financially by their clinic load and financial losses. Commitments to full-time clinical directors and to medical education have not been made here; those commitments give more than other hospitals get in return. That was a big issue for some of our medical directors. Hospitals that have made big investments, though, aren't seen as that strong by the medical school, and our residents aren't much different from theirs. We haven't had that town and gown division that other hospitals have had.

For the most part Larry doesn't understand quality-of-care issues, and he says so, says We must look to our clinical directors. They haven't always understood their role. Larry's put some effort into understanding, but he doesn't "play around in their playpen," which is part of the reason he is successful. He doesn't really understand the trends in this area, and he has given me a free rein. I'm not sure we're doing less well in this area. We could be a lot better. I've tried to push him, and on some things I've made good progress.

The regulators keep messing around with reimbursement and permutations to determine per diems. Just when you figure out one system, they change it. They make us spend a lot of time justifying what we want to do rather than being creative. It's defensive, scrambling to survive reactively rather than proactively. We spend so much time processing, it takes resources that could have been directed toward quality assurance. The process you have to go through to make an empty bed something else is horrendous. Why should you have to prepare a two-inch-thick certificate-of-need proposal and prepare for hearings in order to start a certified home health agency? Start it and see if it survives. Or do that for a 50-bed nursing home? Everything you want to do requiring a certificate of need takes a couple of years or more.

Interview with a Chief of Service

I've known Larry since 195-, when I applied to the staff of the hospital where he used to work. The first great things he did here were, number one, the establishment of the neighborhood health center, one of the first federal grants (the beginning of the turnaround); and, number two, the planning of this new building, a herculean task with many roadblocks he had to overcome—to own it and build it. I was president of the medical staff when we got this building and the $63 million bond issue. I used to go with him and meet with the people involved, in 197-. At the time of the malpractice crisis in 197-, I was working with physicians in the region to meet with the governor. We made 12 recommendations that would have alleviated the crisis, but nothing came of it. I was the chairman of the regional group, and Larry advised me very well. When I told him I was going to get involved with five or six hospitals in the region, he said, Why not get all of them involved? Larry and I are very close on an informal basis. I don't fear him. I speak out and say what I think. I disagree with him probably more than anyone else—to keep some balance, no malice is involved. I'm a member of the steering committee for the merger, and I'm on the board of trustees. Larry is not viewed benignly by the medical staff. He is creative, articulate. He can take any subject and make it come out his way. Larry does not take counsel from anybody. He is headstrong and arbitrary. Once he makes up his mind, nothing can shake him. That has led to accomplishments. No one can argue with success. Now he's surrounded by smart people who can do it too. He doesn't take advice too well.

Everything Larry does is suspect to the medical staff, which is unfair. He says he has their interests at heart, but a lot of them feel the opposite. He's not very political in dealing with this. I don't think he respects them that much. He feels that he is in charge. Friction between administrators and medical staff is a fairly common thing.

He never stops doing things. He has a great imagination. He does his homework.

His is a job that's thankless. You don't get accolades. You work very hard, you get personal gratification, but you don't get complimented by the people around you. The more good things he does, the more criticism he receives. It's not like that in business. He should be given a lot more credit. I wouldn't recommend his job—there's too much harassment, it's too complicated. Larry has a good handle on it. Larry should have been a knight in shining armor when we moved into the new building, but they criticized it. Larry didn't create HMOs or DRGs, but the physicians blame him. They use him as a whipping boy or scapegoat, to vent their frustrations. M.D.'s are frustrated these days. I don't go around defending Larry; I defend him up to a point. I'm sort of in between them and him. I don't criticize him other than to his face.

Larry's made an effort to restore sanity to this neighborhood. It hasn't been that successful. The housing complex, the nursing home, the profit company—probably his greatest quality is his perseverance and endurance, follow-up. He keeps after a problem until he solves it; others would give up. The idea when we built this place was a hospital without walls, "plant a seed and grow a garden." Larry was thinking in terms of economic development, but the neighborhood is still pretty depressed. That was one of the reasons we got this building. If we had wanted to build the hospital in the other local community, it wouldn't have happened.

Socially, I don't see Larry much. He is low-key, he's not into partying. He's conservative. He's happy playing golf and being home. Professionally, I see him once or twice a week and at meetings all the time. We get along pretty well.

He gets things done with his tremendous sense of logical reasoning. He has a way of putting something before a group and making it come out right. He can convince people that what he is saying is correct and for the benefit of the hospital. His first failure was with the merger; I don't know if it was his failure. He is an articulate, logical thinker. I admire that. There are few people who can do that.

Larry always has to have something to do. He can't just sit by. The nursing home is just a matter of waiting. His new venture is the multihospital system. I don't know if it's right or wrong, but it makes sense when he talks about it. Whatever the reasons, it's his latest tack. When the merger waned, he started with another hospital. Minimizing duplication of services will be beneficial medically; it will improve services (all of which we can't have in one institution) that are required for our teaching program—services in which we don't have enough volume to be cost-effective and train residents adequately.

His own abilities are what make him so powerful. He's proven himself to the board without doubt. They don't question him because of his record. I disagree with Larry—I say that we should have a joint conference committee and discuss problems unique to the physician three or four times a year. He says he doesn't want to waste the board's time unless there is something to talk about. He says that board meetings are a proper forum for that. I disagree, because board meetings involve so many other things that medical matters are secondary. Our constitution mentions a joint conference committee. It might make for more understanding if the board could hear first-hand the things we have to say.

In the hospital field Larry doesn't have an equal. He's smarter than any of the others. He knows more. He doesn't make mistakes when he talks. He's direct and convincing. It makes him a better manager. People listen to him.

I like Larry, more as a person than as a manager. He's benign and nice. He's not gregarious or aggressive. He's quiet. We've had little social contact.

I don't think anyone can perform as a CEO in a hospital better than Larry. He irritates people with his smartness. He shoots himself down with his own manipulations. He aggravates people.

Larry hasn't changed much. Before the new building, he wasn't on such firm ground here. They had a different administrator every two years. He was a little humbler. He became more sure of himself, his self-esteem went up and rightly so. He's always been self-assured.

Larry's careful about spending money, relative to others. Medical education is not on the top of his list of priorities. We're a Band-Aid operation. We've always gotten full approval in our service, but I don't know how we do it. We could use help academically in terms of hiring subspecialists part time, but it's difficult to come by. They're conservative in upgrading. At another hospital, they're almost bankrupt the way they spend money. A chief there has three full-time secretaries. Here we have three secretaries for five chiefs. That kind of conservatism keeps us afloat. There's nothing wrong with it. Our reimbursement isn't as good as that of some of the other hospitals either.

All of the administrators here are interested in quality. Larry doesn't have direct input. He leaves it to committees. He has good administrators taking care of it. Our administrators aren't into patient care. They don't make rounds. He doesn't evaluate chiefs relative to quality.

I don't think we would be where we are now without Larry. We might not have a hospital today. We wouldn't be doing all the things we're doing. There are slim pickings to find someone like Larry. For initiative and creativity, he's tops. But he can be arbitrary, not listen to administrative people or take advice. He's single-minded, feeling that his way is the right way. Usually he's right.

Interview with a Nursing Administrator

I started working with Larry in 197- (I've been in the hospital since the 1960s) on planning for the new hospital. He and I and the director of purchasing were the equipment team.

I haven't worked as much with him on nursing issues as on scope of services issues after we moved. People had high expectations and wanted exotic equipment, and I mediated between those who wanted it and Larry. I deal with the COO and not Larry on nursing issues. I know most of the doctors well and gave him a sense of what was going on then.

Larry has really created a unique environment here. He was the catalyst, created something—took a hospital going broke and built a relationship with the community and a unique relationship with the doctors and trustees, to get things done. He is a benevolent dictator. When he came, he told the board he was the professional, to stay out of day-to-day operations (which they had been involved with), or they should tell him to leave. He called the most powerful doctors together and spent a day with them. He told them that if they didn't want him, he would not come. Then being accepted gave him carte blanche to do what he wanted to do. He has a unique position because he's had so many successes. Now people are starting to feel left out [the doctors] and would demand more input.

I think in a business it's more for yourself. A not-for-profit institution is under so much regulation, and more uncertainty as to income, that you can't just raise your prices. It's more difficult, you don't get paid more for doing better. We've got to be more cost-conscious.

Larry created a group in the 1970s that was idealistic, that felt we could change the neighborhood. We're still here, our public relations department is involved with community groups. He has an acute sense of where opportunities are, where we can be involved—getting involved in housing and with senior citizen groups. He was out every night when he first came here, meeting with community groups. He defined health in a broad way, whatever the neighbors needed, at a time when hospitals weren't thinking that way. We were here not to be best at heart surgery, but to do what the neighborhood needed.

I don't interact with him that much, just to say hello. He's out of day-to-day operations. I used to see him for four hours a day, for three or four years.

He has developed about ten people who know him, know what he thinks and have assignments. He would call me in, ask me what I think, and to do what I can. His main thing is creating an environment for the people we are going to work with on a new project, and the staff just does it. He's good at telling stories to create an environment. He tells about our mission, and he tells it in such an interesting way that people sense he is earnest and sincere. This was more so years ago than it is now, and people just took him and gave him what he wanted. He's had very few failures—what's hit him the most is this merger.

He tells me he's trying to create an environment that all of us can leave after he leaves in five or ten years. We need to have a stronger financial base, get some money in the bank from our for-profit corporations, the merger.

His biggest source of power is that everyone knows that the board will go along with whatever he says because he's had a good track record. He's well recognized throughout the country as a prestigious administrator who can get things done. The mayor and governor wanted him to open the new city hospital; a lot of people believe in him.

He went for 10 to 15 years on his having given the medical staff veto power over his coming. They were also helped and encouraged by the things he did—getting a new hospital and equipment—until a few years after we moved here. Now there is more grumbling, which was inevitable. They didn't have much input. We had to move within three years, and we didn't have time to go through a lot of committees. This saved us a lot of money to get it done in three years. Doctors now want more input, whatever that means. They are ambivalent. They like him, but like children who have grown up they depend on him, which they resent. They won't do anything to overthrow him, but if someone else came they'd demand a different setup.

Larry's a leader. He has this charismatic quality that people follow. A manager sets objectives, follows up, and evaluates. Larry doesn't do this in the formal sense, but we all know what his plans are and how we're doing.

He's honest, which is very important, and he's very caring about his staff. He wants his immediate staff close and wants us to do this with our employees, have a close, family-type environment.

I don't think anyone could have done better in providing health care to a neighborhood. The environment in the hospital has changed now. His style needs to allow more participation than he's used to. I don't know that he can change. We need more participatory management. He's trying, but he lacks the patience for committees. He hasn't changed much. These are times for different types of management. It would be better for him to change now, but I don't know if it's possible. He has a quick pickup for new things. It takes others more time to feel a sense of ownership in them.

Larry gave the board and the doctors a choice of whether he was going to be here or not. This gave him the climate that he needed, which makes the difference between him and other managers. Most places aren't as bad as this was when Larry took over. It had gone downhill and was a terrible place and would have closed.

On costs, Larry's made it clear by stating the philosophy of serving our neighbors. We don't do anything that serves a few—open-heart surgery or cancer research—he tells this to everybody.

He built this circle of offices here with clinical and nonclinical officers very close together, unlike other places, where everyone has his or her own kingdom; he didn't want to have that here. He has extremely tight control over the money that goes out. None of us has a real budget. Larry or the COO signs every single check request. If I had a certain amount to spend, I'd have to make hard decisions on what I wanted, so it works the other way too.

On quality of care, Larry doesn't have much to do directly, except for selection of key people. He doesn't get involved in particular problems unless they hit the newspaper. He formed the patient relations department to handle complaints that fall between the cracks, after a serious malpractice case which got into the newspapers.

Larry does have a lot of respect for nurses and the people who work with him. When a chief of surgery demands I fire someone, Larry will not allow that environment to exist. He says it's my responsibility and up to me to decide. So long as he trusts me, he backs me up. It works both ways, if I criticize someone else.

Regarding Ted Grover, CEO of Cleveland Hospital

Interview with the Chairman of the Board

I've worked with Ted Grover since he came into the hospital. I became president in 1970 and was made chairman in 1982. With the merger I wanted Ted to have the title of president.

We work very closely on committee work and the selection of

chairmen of committees and the members of the committees, and the board always approves. We worked closely on the merger and on the reconstruction program. We talk about reimbursement; he knows more about this than I do. I don't feel that the board should be a duplicate of administrative staff. I used to go to seminars and bring back information, and he'd do the same for me. I've seen him grow, and it has been interesting.

You have three groups: trustees, medical staff, and administrators; and it's a little more difficult than in business, working together for the benefit of the hospital. Eastern Airlines has one aim, and you don't have to worry about two or three groups. There lies the seed of real problems. The doctors ganged up on a local administrator and had him fired, and the hospital suffered as a result.

Ted's built up a fine administrative staff, carefully selected, with special skills. He has a real talent for working with people and is well liked by employees. Doctors like him to the extent that they like any administrator. He's approachable, and they can talk with him. He helped to accomplish the merger and was the driving force behind the reconstruction here. He also helped bring about a good feeling with the doctors and trustees. He has been active in the state and city hospital associations and brought our hospital more to the fore. We were always very conservative here. He's brought things to us and shared with others what we do here.

We don't have stated meetings with each other. He's had to be out a good deal. We sometimes spend half an hour, an hour, or longer, at each other's convenience. He has many meetings he has to go to, plus the usual telephone calls.

The trustees are 100 percent behind him. They admire him and respect him. We don't always agree, but we support him. He has a good staff. Ted has a passion for work. He doesn't do things halfway. He's strong, and mentally he's a man who will make decisions. This is often lacking. It's not easy. He thinks things through and makes a decision. So far, it's been right. We hope it continues. We have one of the best administrative staffs in town. They all seem to get along well. Each one helps the other.

Ted has a vision of getting four or five local hospitals together. That two of them wouldn't go along has been disappointing. He's put a lot into this, working with consultants trying to figure out the best way to do things. We miss the old voluntary planning agency. There's no central place that you can go to for help. Ted is active about what we are going to do in the future. Our own finance committee has spent a lot of time on this too.

Ted gets his power from the board. We made him a full trustee last year. We now have a few M.D.'s on the board too.

Ted likes people. He's enthusiastic about what he does. He is thoroughly honest, has a good character, and high integrity. If we don't agree, we're always pleasant about it. He can be very firm, which is important given some of the people that we have to work with.

I rate his performance A+. Ted's a man of his word. When he says he will get something done, he gets it done. He is devoted to the job, patients, employees, and trustees. The employees all like him, and that's saying a lot. He used to be around the hospital more; he regrets not doing that.

He has grown since I first knew him. He's grown more sure of himself. Ted was eager to have the former CEO's job, and some thought that Ted was young, but his predecessor was young too. There is such variety in the job—you must deal with things, different types of people, and sometimes new technology; it's an exciting business.

In influencing costs, Ted and the chief financial officer work very closely together, and Ted works closely with the finance committee. I'm sure there's a lot of waste in a hospital. We changed the man in receiving and stores. We made changes in the head of personnel too. He couldn't deal with unions. We felt bad about it. You must run the hospital for the sick patients, not the employees.

I would rate this hospital as run very well. We get many public patients in the ER who used to go to the municipal hospital. Our ER director is one of 2,000 certified; she's very caring, and our facility is good. We have some very fine chiefs. It's a constant battle to keep the weak points strong. There is turnover. We have difficulty in getting American-trained residents.

Interview with the Vice-President of Medical Affairs

I came here as a chief of service in 196-. In 1970, I was asked to be vice-president of medical affairs. I'm also an associate dean at the medical school.

I try to run my clinical department. I try to balance the professional staff among themselves and their interface with administrators. I'm also chairman of the clinical chiefs here, and we try to interpret and direct the policy of the board of trustees.

I have seen Ted Grover over 20 years, as associate director, CEO, and president of the corporation structure. I deal with him on finance, long-range planning, and development. Today, we deal with managed care and for-profit businesses. The four of us—with the CFO and the COO—seem to get together on this.

We're selling patient care. We're forced to get into a business aspect. The product we're dealing with is human life, which isn't strictly a business. In addition to leading the change and putting us on the map, we must balance cost containment and quality medical care. Heretofore, there wasn't so much concern about cost containment. We've changed from being a purely service organization—we've got to employ business methodology to survive (for example, the development of managed care companies, the syndication of a CT scanner in a local community).

Ted's effected a merger with another hospital. He's been part of the development of a malpractice insurance program that's been quite successful. I think he's an exceptional person—perceptive, intelligent, hard-working. He senses the ebb and flow of things acutely, he's politically astute. He's good-looking.

We see each other ad lib, having working dinners; we interface at a chairman's meeting and at the board of trustees, medical board meetings, corporate executive council (the four of us and two or three others), and we socialize at hospital functions.

He retains the responsibility of the office, but he delegates authority. He keeps the reins tight. The buck stops at his desk, but he delegates authority to get things done. He depends on the people he's chosen; he relies heavily on them.

He's trying to stay afloat now. We are looking at census—recruitment of physicians and direction of patients to the hospital—to association or merger with another hospital. He develops syndications. We are part of the medical school consortium effort; he's active in that.

Ted is tireless and energetic. He perceives relationships among the professional staff well, and he takes the proper stand. There's a group of doctors here who go way back and didn't like the city affiliation; they were opposed to what the administration wanted. Despite that history, Ted acknowledges their existence, interfaces with them, and may help them with a managed company because it's good for the hospital.

He's honest. His word is good. He has social graces. He's not grating or abrasive. He's knowledgeable and hard-nosed. For example, on occasion we have had to ask a physician to leave an administrative post. Other physicians rise against this and threaten, but he says it's got to be done once it's been decided.

A-1, rating his performance! He takes his job extremely seriously, and he knows how to do his job. He's knowledgeable and au courant, for example, about legislation, regulation, and financial matters.

The enlargement of the structure and the pursuit of managed care and syndication force him to delegate authority more. He has the respect of the professional staff (although they try to beat his head in), because he's hard-nosed and knows his business.

Acquiring a mortgage for the merged hospital was a super effort with money so tight and hospitals being cut back. It was not for construction, but for renovation, and they couldn't get a mortgage for rebuilding for a couple of years. Ted was told he couldn't do it. Why waste your energy on this? But he got it.

Regarding cost containment, he is on everybody's back. Do we need this program? Is it cost efficient? We look at the training programs continually. On medical things we convene the chiefs, tell them we need a 5 percent reduction, and ask them to tell us where they will take that from. We've done this with them over and over again.

Ted talks about quality all the time and looks at the people we recruit. He's an elitist in a way. In searching for chiefs, I construct a committee with him, and he or his delegate attends. His input is considered. The search committee makes a choice, directed by Ted and me. This choice is submitted to the medical board more for information (but they say for approval), and then it goes to the board of trustees. In practice, medical board approval has never been a problem. Review of the chief isn't handled so well. We've had to get rid of five or six chiefs. You have to sift reports from the medical staff and then interface with the chief each week. If we agree that this is beyond the pale, we call the chief in and give him a chance, or we don't and make up a separation agreement. If the physician involved is not a chief, we involve the physician and the chairman separately and together.

If you're looking for a prototype of today's CEO, Ted would be it—his knowledge, his work. He is hard-nosed; he doesn't fudge or hedge. He's able to educate his board very well. He interprets for them and makes them understand. Once a year there is a trustees' educational seminar, and he takes great pains with that. Practically, there are many avenues through Ted's office to the board and directly to the board for the physician staff, which has membership on the board and on all the board committees. About 15 of our board members are active and pull their weight, and Ted calls upon them.

We're ending a three-year plan and starting a new one. We have a retreat, invite experts to talk with us, and develop a modus operandi. Our last retreat was 18 months ago. The new plan (we brought in consultants) will have to do with capturing market share. How do we survive, cut costs, and provide quality care? One thought is merger with others.

Interview with the Chief Operating Officer

I work closely with Ted on medical-legal issues, development of professional staff, budget compliance, new program development, joint ventures. We are changing the direction of the corporation—a corporate plan that involves divestiture and for-profit alternative levels of care. This is the future of the corporation, which I am not calling the "hospital."

Against a background of barriers—tax, reimbursement, hospital regulations—general acute hospital care is not financially viable in this state, given the population we serve; you create an infrastructure of governance, initiative, and control that allows you to do for-profit and not-for-profit things. We created that structure. Currently we have an imaging center, an industrial medicine company; soon we shall have a pharmacy, durable medical equipment, and intensive home care; further down the line, we will go into cardiac rehabilitation and skilled nursing home facilities. This requires management, labor law, and tax people. At the same time, we are watching our regular activities and how the new activities will fit with them.

The irrationality of this business—you've got a reimbursement system that doesn't pay you for what you've got to do, you've got a quality assurance system that asks you to do more. You operate constantly not knowing who your customer is: Is it the employer, who adds costs to his product by adding health services? The patient, who expects everyone to be friendly and nice? The physician, who wants the latest equipment and the most supportive nurses? Labor unions, who throw their entire aspirations regarding career development, salary, and professional prestige in the CEO's lap? The CEO has to deliver. At any moment, night or day, the slightest procedural mistake can harm a patient.

Ted's built a new hospital in a regulatory environment where that's "impossible." He's created a vision of the future that's understood by clinical leadership, trustees, and his management team. He's created a spirit that attracts good people, which is why the hospital runs so well. There was a moratorium on capital projects. There was a series of technical reviews of the hospital's financial viability and debt feasibility that he had to go through for both hospital buildings which no one else had done.

I interact with him in three ways: (1) private meetings, which last from five minutes to an hour (I take a systematic list to these meetings); (2) council meetings, where he sits at the head of the table with me and my peers, we talk about things that need reconciling or that crisscross our responsibilities, and he reports to us on outside advocacy or on things that he takes responsibility for; (3) at a local Italian restaurant, where we think about new ideas, once a month, sometimes more, or after a meeting. He has an aptitude for visualizing the practical steps almost immediately, insisting upon them in the same moment. He can listen to abstractions and say, What you need to do is 1-2-3-4! He has energy, charisma, and a mercurial management style. You've got four minutes to develop a project, then he's into socializing. He would call you into question if you take longer. He has a focused, practical style, with a bias towards action.

I think he's always trying to create an institution that is appropriate for the 1990s—diversified, for-profit activities; merger with key hospitals to create a systems approach; focus on marketing and community relations; and managed care, integrating hospital care with nursing homes, home care, and other programs that will feed the hospital and be fed by it.

He spends an incredible amount of his emotional energy making the payroll, handling the citation from the state health department when it comes in, pulling two doctors apart or the state and the hospital together.

His tenure is a source of power. He was associate director for operations; his years of delivering to people have given him remarkable credibility, from department heads to clinicians. His personality galvanizes people's spirit around an issue, so technical support is provided enthusiastically—you want to please him. He receives a lot of support from trustees—I've never met a man with more board support. He turned an insurmountable, unviable Victorian building into a brand new building with 92 percent occupancy. He never takes a problem to anyone without a solution, even if he's at the center of the problem.

He's not ponderous. He doesn't want to hear the statistics, but what the statistics tell us. He tries to minimize analysis. He has an unbelievable knack for how the different parties at interest will view what he's about to do. He's not a plodder. He works in incredible spurts of activity, and then he goes fishing.

He gives and demands respect. (For example, in the midst of a meeting full of important people, he will interrupt discussion to thank the dietary worker who brought the coffee.) He trades on personal loyalty rather than facts, figures, or job assignments—they don't always correspond to the organizational chart.

His performance is one of the best that I've ever seen. He works in a system in which he is allowed to carry out management discretion rather than be involved in governance, oversight, and budget offices.

I see a man in transition. He comes from a background of operations, a tangible world to work in. Now all the tangible things are basically delegated, and he must take on statesman functions of advocacy and policy. In times of stress, he reverts to the solace of giving orders and seeing something done.

He influences costs directly: he orders austerity programs, sets goals for reductions (by some percentage), and expects programmatic refinements and developments to deliver results. I've already been through three of those. He's encouraged his counterpart in medical affairs to oversee clinical judgments, such as use of ancillaries. What present reductions are ordered is a judgment call, based on finance department opinion as to what revenues we can expect and what he thinks is flexible.

Ted is quite specific in guiding quality assurance and risk management. He has remained directly involved in these. He listens personally to reports on medical malpractice cases. The medical affairs committee reviews data on quality assurance processes. He has replaced an executive who was doing a good job because his growth potential was limited, a very young person. He creates an atmosphere in which people know that cleanliness, friendliness, respect for smokers and nonsmokers, what the grounds look like, people lounging around in surgical garb in the neighborhood will get his direct comments or correction. He wants to know if the graffiti haven't been cleaned up.

There are lots of ways my job can be wrenching and emotional—hours of work and then disappointment when I've done my best work and get attacked. In almost a two-minute encounter, he gives me the feeling of his energy, support, and backing. I get more out of his personality than almost anything he does.

Interview with the Chief Financial Officer

I've been director of finance and vice-president for finance since 197-. I work with Ted on the serious general financial problems we experience from time to time. The most recent problem is reimbursement rates: (1) the mortgage applications from each hospital; (2) our malpractice insurance program, which is time-consuming (we are affiliated with six other hospitals and their doctors, and this is a $60 to $70 million program); (3) merger; (4) general financial issues that come up at budget and rate approval times. We also work on physician contract issues and the financial end of union contracts (this has diminished since 198-).

As part of the merger, we became subject to a special section of the reimbursement code. We've taken exception to the state reimbursement rates and are trying to convince them they are wrong. The main issues relate to calculation of penalties we felt were inappropriate about length of stay—we didn't have the evidence until the end of 1982, but it still has been a few years. We try to act reasonably, to the degree that we can. We meet with them, lay out our case, and decide what we can and cannot agree on. Ted goes when we discuss principles. He's got a good relationship with the people there and is effective. They don't do everything that he would like, but they believe what he says.

In this business you're not always in control of your own destiny. It's such a heavily regulated industry. While you may have the best intentions, sometimes you can't do the right thing to produce a positive result because of crazy regulations. You just learn to live with regulators and legislators—to understand their point of view and their agendas and to try to extract the best possible compromise from a situation.

The key internally is getting a competent staff and realizing that you must delegate. Other hospital CEOs are reluctant to delegate, and that's a shortcoming.

Key things Ted has done include: number one, the merger; number two, the rebuilding of the hospital site and the approval to renovate the other hospital's site; number three, his ability to work well in the political and legislative areas and with a wide variety of people—to the point where he's become a respected spokesman for the hospital and the industry. He has a fine relationship with our local government, which has helped us obtain approval to rebuild the hospital that we merged with.

Ted's also worked well with people in Washington to get the mortgage approved. We engaged a Washington lobbyist and got in touch with Senator [Orrin] Hatch and met with Secretary [Margaret] Heckler's number one deputy, who was instrumental in getting the project approved by the Department of Health and Human Services, acting for the Department of Housing and Urban Development. Heckler's staff had rejected our applications, mostly for financial reasons, and we got this decision overturned. We convinced them that their interpretation of the facts was erroneous and that certain facts weren't being considered. That program was designed specifically for hospitals which couldn't get financing elsewhere, like us.

We have no specialized, formalized meetings. We talk sporadically, go to certain meetings together, and spend a great deal of time on mortgage applications and the merger.

Ted delegates and has brought together a good team that he has confidence in. He will talk to people and resolve matters when that's warranted. We're experiencing serious cash problems and are trying to work out longer payments with certain vendors, one of which is the union. Ted worked out something with such a leader by picking up the phone. He was the only one who could have made that call and got that reaction from that particular person.

He sees the necessity for us to align or merge with a bigger system in order to be better able to function in what he sees the environment to be, when volume is shrinking and downsizing will occur. We may not be able to function, given our financial problems, otherwise. We need to get a more solid base, to contract in certain areas and expand in others.

He is able to convince other people and our physician staff that what we're doing is the right way to do it. He articulates his position very well. The people who work with him, including enough physicians, feel that he is capable and that what he is doing is correct. They have faith in his ability. He's got an excellent rapport with the trustees, who are supportive.

He is concerned with the individual. Other superiors haven't been so concerned. Three-and-one-half years ago, I had a stroke and was out of work for three or four months; Ted was very supportive and told me not to worry. His support was helpful. He's not afraid to make tough decisions. With respect to the merger, it became clear that a VP of medical affairs at the other hospital had to go, and Ted wasn't afraid to make that decision.

Ted is outgoing and personable. We get along extremely well. We've had fun and been through tough times together too.

I give him an excellent rating for his performance. When Ted took over as executive director, I questioned in my own mind whether he had sufficient maturity to get a major commitment to rebuild. But he stepped in and has done an excellent job, representing us within the association and with local government and legislative people.

He delegates more now, which is a natural evolution for that kind of position. You're almost forced to do that.

Ted has a good feel for the cost of what we're doing. When he becomes convinced that we're spending too much or doing something we shouldn't be doing, he speaks up. We've had six or more austerity programs to balance our operations. He's not a spendthrift, certainly. The main causes of our financial problems: there was a big census downturn in 198-, HMO admissions did not materialize, and at the merged hospital physicians who had been using it as a secondary hospital could now use the hospital of their choice because of falling censuses. Things are improving now. The DRG system is a positive factor for us over the first months. We anticipate breaking even, depending on dealings about rates.

Ted influences quality in terms of what we're spending and what programs we implement with what professional staff. He is committed to quality care and medical education. He tries to obtain the best salaried staff he can. Programs have been implemented that have added to quality.

Another major accomplishment was the disaffiliation from the municipal hospital. We had a medical program for an 800- to 900-bed hospital. We lived through six false starts on its closure. We've been able to maintain the educational programs. This was behind the merger: we moved the full-time physicians, many of them, there. We had 400 to 500 people shared with the municipal hospital, most of them physicians. Some we absorbed, some we let go, and we reduced the size of the training programs.

Regarding Sam Woodrow, CEO of Wilson HMO

Interview with the Chief Financial Officer

I've been here since May 1973. Sam came in August of 1978. I've worked with him on buying the [medical] groups' facilities, regionalizing the groups and making them full-time, and converting to an HMO. Now we're working on the expansion programs—inside our service area we are adding facilities and capacity, and outside our service area we are making new starts and acquiring other plans and possibly starting up IPA models.

Health care is a very regulated industry—and health organizations function in a very political environment. The general public understands and perceives the need for health care. You always find the politicians there (for example, at any opening of a new center). It puts us in a goldfish bowl. Issues are resolved more slowly, and we get involved with the political structure (for example, when you talk about closing a center, not only is it a fiscal matter, it is also a matter of convincing politicians and consumers that it's necessary). Your production is your doctors, so you have to find ways to work with physicians who are independent and don't have a real sense of what the consumer wants. They look at health care as treating sick patients, not as treating the buyer in the way he or she wants to be treated.

Key things that Sam has done: first, he made the groups full-time (he changed the delivery system). Second, he convinced the city government to buy the HMO package (they had to pay more money and give members less choice). Third, he took a provincial plan and broadened its outlook to expand into new regions and new markets with new products. He felt the delivery system was faulty in that we didn't capture the hospital savings as other HMOs do. His philosophy is that, unless you grow, you die as your population ages.

The corporation has grown fiscally; revenues are up from $130 million to over $500 million. The surplus is much stronger. He's provided a motivation, a sense of vigor and excitement that didn't exist before. Rarely a day passes that I don't meet with him on several issues, for periods ranging from 15 minutes to several hours.

He has the management team work by objectives. He tries to establish goals and policies that are clear to everyone. Then officers are responsible for implementing them. To start this out, you've got to convince the board that these goals are in the corporate interest. The previous board didn't see the urgency of making these changes. People were getting health care services, and the board couldn't make the leap from fee-for-service M.D.'s in private practice to full-time M.D.'s in new facilities. They weren't attuned to what was happening in health care in the rest of the country. First he convinced the board that we ought to be willing to spend money to get a full-time system. He had to convince the medical groups that it was in their interest to go full time. It took four years to complete the whole process—18 months to convince the board and the medical groups. We negotiated with our medical groups, which took quite a long time, and slowly we convinced every group. Arguments: number one, we would provide fiscal incentives to take care of them financially; number two, we would buy their facilities at a reasonable price; number three, Wilson was out of step with regard to HMOs elsewhere. We convinced the groups to sell their medical facilities to the plan and to take a small down payment with a 30-year mortgage. We did the whole process in steps, so we didn't have to make all the payments in the same year (putting them on a full-time basis). We also got them to agree to take original cost on their centers, which we defined as net depreciated value plus accumulated depreciation.

Sam sees that the resultant health care players will be bigger and national in scope. We must relate to mostly national accounts, independently or with others. The consumer is no longer satisfied with traditional health care packages—employers will be more stringent, so employees will want to buy different packages. We must be more flexible with consumers. The next five to ten years will be competitive with regard to price. We must find ways of delivering health care in a much more efficient way. We're going into the preferred provider programs in July—we shall offer them first to public and commercial accounts. The consumer will sign up and get services at no cost if he or she gets care through our centers; if the consumer goes outside for services, the plan will pay 80 percent and the consumer will pay a 10 percent higher premium (the consumer gets all hospitalization if certified). The customer gets a choice on top of the HMO package for a price. Sam has also concluded that the IPA model is acceptable to consumers so far, so we shall market this outside our service area.

Sam has a very convincing personality. He formulates something in a way people understand and can convince them of the wisdom of doing it his way. His reputation, that he's built up over the years, gives him credibility and stature. He makes a logical presentation of issues. He is a man of his word and won't promise what he can't perform.

Most CEOs are hard-working, are demanding of their people, and have strategies that are well thought out, depending on their success. Sam is a good communicator. You know where you stand. You know what your goals and objectives are. You're given an opportunity to participate in decisions. A lot of CEOs will make decisions and have you implement them. Sam's good at getting everyone involved. He is very considerate of his staff. (For example, I know of people here who have problems, physical or emotional, and he's helped them where others would have given up.) He's more accessible than many CEOs. He's remarkably open and frank.

He doesn't look like a CEO. He likes most of the things that others like. He's a little more reflective. He's always into new facets of health care and associations of people that stimulate him. He's also very committed to equal opportunity and affirmative action. This is reflected in the staff of Wilson. And he's been able to get good results. This reflects a social commitment.

I would rate him triple A or excellent. That doesn't mean there are certain jobs I would necessarily give him (for example, in operations). His real interests are in planning and marketing. He has less interest in mechanics.

His track record has been superb. He has accomplished here things which others couldn't accomplish.

Overall, he hasn't changed. He's a little more understanding of the timing required to accomplish things. He's developed more patience and persistence. He's more willing to accept some defeats in order to accomplish larger objectives.

He's very, very insistent on keeping totally up-to-date on his mail. He's very conservative on perquisites. He doesn't want any employees to spend money frivolously on seminars, travel, and things like that. He's very concerned that proper staff work and good analysis have been done on anything that goes out of Wilson. He's very particular about how things are worded.

On containing costs, he mainly preaches, As nice as some things sound, they're not worth it in the premium. He stresses efficiency and hard work to the doctor—productivity and not treating patients when they don't need it, or spending money and not accomplishing anything. He gets involved directly in negotiations with the medical groups and at the tail end of the budget. He's probably better informed than most CEOs. (For example, he was directly involved in reducing average length of stay at our own hospital. He put in a bonus arrangement with our medical groups, and it's worked—the average has dropped from above eight days per stay to below six.)

He has had the most extensive quality control mechanisms put in place of any of the prepaid group practices. The M.D.'s in each group audit the practices of other doctors in the group (5 to 10 percent of charts) relative to established standards. Then there is peer review from the central organization, which reviews the audits and the standards. In the medical groups, the audit committee either educates or gets rid of the substandard M.D. As a result, medical staff performance has been improved. The staff know someone is looking at them, and they will therefore document care better. Sam was directly involved in seeing that it was done. He gets statistics and asks questions in this area. He has also been instrumental in getting information on consumer attitudes and on attitudes towards Wilson.

Interview with an Administrator

I've been in the HMO business since 197-. In October of 197-, I came to Wilson as executive assistant to the president and have served in a multitude of capacities.

I work with Sam on issues related to our competitive standing—what do we do and how do we do it to put ourselves in the best strategic position (for example, the failed merger and patient relations program and how this is packaged)? I also work heavily in the areas of negotiating mergers and acquisitions, expansion, and new products. I act as a sounding board. Sam will say to me, How does this play? (talking about reorganization of the corporation and who's capable of what kind of job, for example). And I work in the political arena.

Without understanding the history, culture, and environment of Wilson, you're doomed to fail—history and an appreciation of the fact that Wilson had many defects and flaws, but there were valid historical reasons why. The plan was underplanned and underfinanced when it started, piggybacked on physicians who were entitled to say that Wilson was supported on the backs of their service. They were paid, but not enough.

Culture and environment—you must accept the premise that Wilson is an institution in this city. There are linkages with power forces here that cannot be ignored. Compromises and concessions have to be made: for example, when we converted city employees to the HMO, we agreed to let them go outside the system for a year or two and we would pay the bill. Sam overlooks episodic anecdotal evidence of medical group insensitivity in dealing with members, because the groups are still grappling with rapid change in their lives. We take the long view. If behavior is in the right direction and if they understand the basic premises, positive behavior will become the rule rather than the exception.

Reorganizing Wilson so that we can function as an organization has been Sam's paramount accomplishment. He's been able to do this through consensus rather than bloodshed. He's been able to turn the image of Wilson around. Now we are considered an organization with integrity, and we are seen as trying to do a good job. Sam switched the authority and responsibility to central management and has gotten it accepted (it had been all over the place—there were power brokers who were quasimanagers, everything was muddy). He's been able to attract and build a competent management team that wants to do a good job. Before, managers came here to die.

Sam was able to obtain a solid understanding of the history and culture of the organization before he took the job; when on the job he touched base with everyone he could and got a lot of opinions from everyone. He then put himself in the skin of those whose behavior he wanted to change—negotiation, not coercion, was the key to success (he lacked the power levers then anyway). Sam was able to devise ways and means of getting various constituents to agree to changes; he devised strategies for allowing them to see changes as in their interest. For example, we didn't tell the 26 medical groups they had to be nine groups, but we financed combined larger groups at a higher rate (because they did extra things). In the same way we provided financing to buy out their facilities and gave them assurances that it was in their interest. It's less that he's a wizard than that he has a good sense of timing in terms of what you can and cannot do.

Sam, basically, did what his predecessor was trying to do many years previously. For example, in one locale we have three medical groups instead of one; there is no reason for that. If we had pushed too hard in that area, however, we might have lost some of the other medical group mergers. We didn't have enough levers to force that merger, so we backed off. We did end up with fewer than the six or seven medical groups that had been in that area.

He did what he did because he believed that we could not be efficient and prepaid unless we followed more closely the genetic code of Kaiser: no system without a functioning health plan and no health plan without the ability to determine the system's facilities, organization, and direction. Previously we were more like an insurance company. We could not finance what we wanted to do without capturing the hospital savings. We could not be competitive without large full-time groups.

Sam finds challenge challenging and maintenance of an organization unchallenging. To take an organization from struggle to success was attractive. At that time in the industry it was either fee-for-service or group practice. There were no multilines of business. He figured out the way we should be organized, set his priorities so the dominoes would fall. We needed to go HMO; then we could finance the groups and buy their facilities.

Interaction with Sam varies, depending on what's hot—it ranges from intense to minimal. Sam gets things done: there is general agreement that Sam has integrity. If you are part of his team, you feel you're not being set up. If you're not part of his team at a given moment, you don't feel that you have been simply used and discarded. If people trust you, and they do trust Sam, it helps get things done.

Sam's priorities now are (1) iron out the rest of the glitches in the system; (2) raise the esprit de corps of the organization, the sense of pride and professionalism (Kaiser has done an excellent job on this— the employees' sense of pride in the organization contributes heavily to its success); and (3) do what's necessary to be one of the survivors when the national shakeout is over. This will take more than a local HMO; whether regional or national, you will need a lot of members, money, to be price-sensitive, and you need several lines of business. How do you do that without losing your integrity and sense of social purpose?

His predominant source of power is his ability to understand the tenor of the times, to present proposals that keep Wilson strong and to win consensus without damage to the organization. Managers in some other settings are bulls in a china shop; they accomplish as much but with enmity as the fallout. Sam is able to see the broader picture, accept that the world isn't perfect, you've got to give to get. He is able to compromise on issues without compromising his personal integrity.

I'd give him an A for performance. He accomplished what others said couldn't be done. It was accomplished without losing anyone we wanted to keep.

Sam has changed a lot in the past year or two. He understands that our world is far more complex. It's no longer just prepaid versus fee-for-service practice. He is no longer capable of having the only answer to a problem. He's more receptive to input and advice. For example, I was able to talk with him about our strategy for expansion—about doing IPAs upstate, expanding to new states, and creating new product lines such as PPOs.

People approach me to see how something will play with Sam—to try out new ideas with me, to see if Sam will be receptive, and to see if they can recruit me as an advocate for what they want to accomplish.

The primary way he influences the cost of care is by facilitating prepaid multispecialty group practice, which saves on hospitalization and takes advantage of economies of scale. The other major way is that Sam has initiated incentives to foster cost-effective behavior—for example, the hospital bonus for physicians who are below the target on hospitalization, with a limit on the upside for individual physicians. At first, seven of nine groups were getting nothing, so he backed off the formula and gave partial rewards for getting closer to the target. This has enhanced medical groups' support for more hospital monitoring.

The first step in quality assurance was getting multispecialty group practice; that way you get peer review and true self-policing, which is happening. Groups are now interdependent on Wilson. A full-time physician in the Wilson system now has his or her success tied to Wilson's performance. It's starting to happen that, if a physician is not performing according to our standards, other physicians understand it will affect their own economic survival and self-esteem. This does a lot to enhance quality, as does the strong quality assurance program we have implemented.

Sam has been trying to institute quality of performance. We're building a management team and a code of ethics. Also, you can't allow Wilson to be kicked around if you work here.

Interview with Another Administrator

I came to Wilson from another state in 198-. I had first worked with Sam many years ago. I was both marketing director and executive director at a Wilson subsidiary. We ran a holding action and transferred functions as we could to the main office. Our staff went down to two people. We still have coordination problems (for example, we have a four-step rate in our state, as do most of our major accounts; there is a three-step rate in our home state).

Sam is my last resort. I'm careful how I approach him. You don't bring him things you can solve yourself. We don't let our friendship interfere with business. We see each other socially three or four times a year, and I never discuss business issues then. Sam is a hard taskmaster. You must have your facts very clear. He goes right to the heart of the issue. I've come to Sam six to eight times over this period. For example, I've seen him about marketing issues. The senior vice-president in the main office was responsible for marketing issues in our subsidiary, and we weren't getting the attention we needed. It took time to get a full-time marketing director, about nine months.

A second example is that of a center that wouldn't allow us to grow. We and the facilities staff in the main office chose a new site; Sam was involved in the site selection. The new center, 20,000 square feet, is up and running now in a different community. The old center has stayed flat at 8,200 members; we opened with 300 members in the new center and now have 6,200 members there.

What Sam has been able to do is (1) surround himself with trustworthy and knowledgeable people; (2) grasp the overall needs of the organization very quickly; and (3) set in place a course of action after discussion with everyone around him. He's not arbitrary, and he involves everyone in the establishment of goals. He is goal-oriented, which is nice because you understand what you're trying to do. He gives you tasks and expects them to be completed: Take care of it and don't screw it up. His door is open, but the task is there and you're supposed to handle it. It took a long time and a lot of patience when we transferred functions from here to the main office; people in the main office thought, This isn't the way we have done things. We had to get down to operating on a break-even basis.

The board is different here. At another HMO where we worked together the board was business-oriented and more intellectual; it understood the marketplace and what had to be done. Here at Wilson there are conflicts between unions whose members are served by the plan, which gives the board a parochial rather than a global view. Sam had to be concerned with the board's direction, to get it to go from medical care delivery to HMO, to be at risk for the hospital side. To Wilson members, this reduced their freedom of choice. To get the board to move to an HMO was difficult; so was getting it to decide to move medical groups to full-time.

Key for us has been his getting the board to assist Wilson in our state as part of the organization and getting it to fund us, opening members' eyes to see that Wilson has a larger scene to play in and to continue to move it in a different direction (this has been important). The board now accepts that we may have to do things differently in this state to succeed in the market. To stand still is to fall behind.

Sam gets things done by asking. There's no such comment as, I can't do it. If you need help, he'll supply it. He expects it to be done and therefore you do it—and do it without disruption to other people.

He is determined to make this the best organization in the country—to make it equal to or better than Kaiser's organization—not in size but in stature. Kaiser's a well-run business organization. We wear our hearts on our sleeves more than necessary. We became a public whipping boy, and it's not justified. And he's correct. There was a lack of pride here which Sam has changed, but it's difficult to overcome. They always used to make excuses about everything, and we really weren't bad at all.

His power comes from two areas: (1) his knowledge of everything that deals with medical care and of HMOs in particular and (2) his ability to get things done. He is able to identify problems that have to be solved to accomplish an end result. For example, when we opened the second center I wanted to shut down the first center and open a new one someplace else. Sam said we couldn't afford to have two faucets open—the old center and the new center are both losing money. If we closed the old center, we should strengthen the new center before opening another one. He said we should put all our eggs in one basket until the new second center gets into the black.

He's more human, able to discuss issues not on a power basis. He doesn't flaunt his power or beat you up with it. He's willing to listen to what you have to say. He's demanding and expects detail, but he will explain his reasons. He's sensitive to what his word was if you are following through on something. He doesn't want problems brought to him as problems, but as resolved issues. Others would say, Take care of it, and threaten you. As long as you give your best effort, Sam doesn't want to give you more than you can do or expose your weaknesses in front of other people.

He has an undying loyalty to people he's been involved with. It's phenomenal. He'll put up with a lot of incompetency because of loyalty to people. He has a strong feeling about the inequities of the social system to minorities and wants to respond to those as much as possible. He was the first in this field to put a woman in the top marketing position, for example. You'll see it on his staff.

I'd rate him an 8 out of 10. He surrounds himself with people he is comfortable with and who can do the job. He's got a good handle on determining people's abilities and using them to the fullest. He hangs on to incompetent people too long. There is no fast action on this kind of matter.

He's not nearly as naive as he used to be. Sam had stars in his eyes. He surprises me in his ability to read people. I was away from him for ten years. He became much more confident and directed.

Sam has taken this organization from what it was to a prepaid group practice plan that rivals Kaiser in every feature—buying out facilities and making them consistent, keeping the organization moving forward during a time of transition. When we go out to talk to people, the reaction is often negative. Physicians are now committed to this organization and its members.

He wants Wilson in this state to lose as little money as possible, so long as we can be effective. He expects us to get the best deal from hospitals. For example, if we are high performers with DRGs, it should be reflected in our deal. He questions areas of our financial report at every board meeting. As to financing of our facilities—we were going to do it through banks, but we did it through the state health authority because it cost less, even though it delayed completion of our center.

He doesn't really get involved in quality assurance. Our medical group must conform to the same policies as groups in our home state. He's told the medical director in the home state that's what he wants (she used to be medical director here). On service, he only gets involved if someone sends a letter.

It's difficult to know the pressures he's under on an ongoing basis. He doesn't really tell you. You know they are there. His position is unique—it's quasi-governmental because of Wilson's history and membership. A person who's running a business doesn't have to so respond. He's sensitive to damaging information in the newspapers. Corruption in the city has made him doubly concerned.

Interview with the Medical Director at the HMO where Sam Woodrow Formerly Worked

A few months into the program, it became obvious we were having problems. The board didn't have the time or the desire to look, we needed change quickly, we looked internally, and Sam was selected as CEO. We had two medical groups in our facility. In March 197-, the two groups were merged. I took over as medical director in 197-. Our HMO is different from the normal medical world in that insurance is not separate from delivery—we set our own goals, strategies, and priorities, see to it that it is our program, our values that emerge. The distinctions of what we were responsible for were blurred among the managing group. We were a small group who drew on each other for support and ideas. It's different now. We shared decision making. Sam's responsibilities were focused on finance, marketing, personnel, institutional and contractual relationships, systems. Mine were in recruiting clinical staff, developing facilities, and care arrangements and relationships with hospitals.

You have to understand what it takes to be successful in the marketplace (competition then was more focused on the local Blues plan), what it takes to manage an organization. None of us on the medical side had that management experience.

Within a fairly brief period of time, Sam restored the confidence of key people that we were being led and had direction, that although the odds were against us we had a chance to succeed.

He had to revise the marketing strategy. It took three years to accomplish what was necessary, moving away from dependence on the Blues. He led the plan in the direction of taking the risk. In year one we saved $750,000 and did the job better.

He had good judgment about people, who ought to staff the key positions in the organization. He saw when it wasn't going very well in an area and then bit the bullet and made critical personnel decisions. He could define what the organization needed and make the right replacement.

He took responsibility but could share this to make others feel that they were critical to success. His relationship with physician leaders was outstanding. He was respected and trusted; he had authority in areas where we needed it. He was able to create an atmosphere in which we who were leaders believed in the long-term worth of what we were doing, that new ground was being broken, that we had the potential to make a big difference. People were willing to engage and struggle to resolve differences of opinion. He had good instincts about what was not going well. You trusted his instincts and judgments based on his presentation. The physicians had strong institutional ties with a different culture than fee-for-service, which helped.

He developed a strong relationship with the leadership of the board, who were inexperienced in health care but of enormous stature and who knew they were in trouble. Within a few months, they had confidence that Sam knew how to lead or would get help when help was needed. The red ink that flowed then should not be underestimated. The stupid, ill-conceived, and uninformed decisions we made in those early days would fill a big book. How do you manage a tight ship? We didn't know how to respond when clinicians wanted more staff to do well.

He forced the issue of getting the two medical groups into one. He lived with that two-group setup for 18 months. He would continuously point out the problems it was causing, that decisions took too long. It was based on assumptions, no longer valid, that the two groups would be based in two facilities. In the first few months, you felt you were working for the this-or-that hospital and had been assigned to the HMO. It took a while for people to change their identifications. Paychecks were changed to HMO when the groups were merged. He never made it feel like a power play. His attitude was, We are all in agreement that we want to survive, and this decision-making structure gets in the way. He forced the issue, not the exact timing or form, but its resolution and direction.

The executive committee of the board was his source of power. The dean and associate deans, who empowered him to be their representative—they worked together closely. There was this quality of believing in what we were doing and wanting an effective leader. When he came on the scene and demonstrated these qualities, the situation fit with what he brought to it. This went a long way in empowering him. He had a remarkable presence. He made us feel that the boat was being guided—partly through his political sense, his common-sense judgment and ability to work with people, to get them to come together and work effectively.

I think he had the feeling that the clinicians didn't have high enough in their value system (1) how much members who made only $12,000 or $15,000 a year had to pay to belong and (2) making the visit feel like a humanly enjoyable experience for the patient. (From the viewpoint of the physician, doing a good job was diagnosis and treatment.) How closely identified with the teaching hospitals can this program be over the years? (In 197- we dealt with it by getting our own hospital; in 198- expanding our hospital was more expensive than tying back to a teaching hospital.) He would have liked to have seen us more productive, cost-conscious, making every visit feel right to the patient.

We had a genial bond. I was fresh out of residency, in my first management job. He was new to the city, supposedly in charge of marketing, and the ship was about to go under. There was a closeness about the working relationship and the feeling about it. Other managers have more purely intellectual, analytical abilities. He has more ability to separate the wheat from the chaff—deciding when and where to move and what it takes to move, managing the human enterprise. I want Sam to set the agenda for the analysis and to pick the right analyst for where the organization is trying to go. His toughest decision here, which he handled masterfully, was the separation from

Blue Cross. We weren't risk takers; we were closely tied to the medical school. Sam said, We're going into the insurance business regardless of Blue Cross's $8 million in reserves. There were too many things we needed under our control that we couldn't control in that relationship (for example, each change in benefits had to go through the Blue Cross benefit committee).

He's straight, honest. I enjoyed coming to work with him, although we were in conflict 30 percent of the time. Our disagreements were related to the bigger context rather than being translated into personal conflict.

A little slow off the mark—Sam came with limited experience, but he was a very fast learner. If Sam wasn't the major reason, it was because of him and the dean that we survived. He was effective and did a first-rate job and made us feel the organization was going the right way.

On cost containment, in the early days he would say, This is what must be according to the budget. The delivery system was split, with M.D.'s reporting to the medical director and other workers to the executive director. It was tough then to make trade-off decisions. Chiefs in specialties had difficulties. Now there is a medical director in each center who is responsible for budget and personnel in that center.

On quality assurance, his focus was on service. With respect to technical quality, he assumed that the medical leadership would take care of it. He focused attention on the importance of service by his selection of managers, by developing training programs emphasizing those features.

Effective managers empower those under them to define and deal with problems, enabling the managers to do the broader, strategic planning.

6.

Observed Activities and Episodes of Work

In this chapter I show the activities and episodes of work I observed for each of the four CEOs on a Monday, Tuesday, and Wednesday (each CEO was actually followed for five days). Then, for each CEO, activities are grouped to focus upon one episode of work spanning the three-day period.

Activities and episodes for each day are listed chronologically. Some of the episodes include one activity, others more than one. An *activity* is an interaction between the CEO and one or more others on a particular topic; an *episode* is a group of activities on the same subject. Episodes and activities are categorized by time as follows: brief (under 10 minutes), intermediate (11 to 30 minutes), long (31 to 60 minutes), and very long (over 60 minutes).

The episodes spanning the three-day period involve from 4 to 11 activities. They are on the following topics: the response of Washington Medical Center to competitor organizations offering managed care; the terminating of Van Buren Hospital's sharing of OB-GYN services with another hospital; complaints about a chief of service at Cleveland Hospital; and recruitment of a chief operating officer for a Wilson HMO subsidiary.

Tim George, CEO of Washington Medical Center

Monday (12 hours)

Activities and Episodes	Time Spent
1. Trustee requests the name of a doctor for a friend; CEO refers him to COO.	Brief
2. Other CEO calls, indicating that his institution will not be part of a third organization's affiliation network for managed care. George discusses managed care with M.D. job applicant, with associate administrator, and with full-time internist.	Brief
3. CEO participates with the dean in review of performance of a clinical chairman.	Intermediate
4. CEO participates with the dean in review of performance of a second clinical chairman.	Intermediate
5. CEO conducts job interview with a physician whose primary appointment would be in the department of medicine.	Long
6. CEO calls director of nursing in response to a question about the number of nursing students in the hospital.	Brief
7. CEO indicates support for a development project, in response to an M.D. request, and communicates this to the director of development.	Brief
8. CEO agrees to give blood.	Brief
9. CEO requests from PR some publicity for a laudatory article on a clinical chairman, with whom this is cleared.	Brief
10. CEO agrees to a request from a clinical chief to review space plans in a new building.	Brief
11. CEO is requested by a trustee to facilitate admission of a patient to a nursing home affiliated with the hospital. CEO follows up by meeting with social worker and by calling the nursing home. The admitting physician is not available but will call back. CEO calls the trustee back.	Intermediate
12. CEO is told that a study on operating room efficiency is proceeding.	Brief

13. CEO informs another hospital CEO of the search for his successor. CEO discusses succession with VP for human resources.   Brief

14. CEO is informed that M.D.'s wife is pleased with award M.D. has received.   Brief

15. CEO is informed that an assistant administrator is working on do-not-resuscitate guidelines.   Brief

16. CEO asks how lawyers are dealing with development of a hospital property in the face of resistance from an historic preservation group.   Brief

17. CEO is informed that an assistant administrator is responding to a state health department investigation of a complaint about emergency services.   Brief

18. CEO is told by community relations staff about relocation plan related to sale of a hospital property to a private developer; CEO will visit the building into which tenants will be relocated.   Intermediate

19. CEO is told about VIP (the brother of a potential large donor) who has been admitted; CEO will visit.   Brief

20. Physician complains to CEO that a new building obstructs the view of a plaque for a previously honored physician; CEO will follow up.   Brief

21. CEO is told about locals who wish to sell a third property; he asks for more information.   Brief

22. CEO tells donor that room which donor paid to refurbish is ready for viewing.   Brief

23. Lawyer requests CEO's permission to attend an educational conference; CEO grants request.   Brief

24. CEO is informed that a second VIP is a patient in the emergency services area; CEO will visit.   Brief

25. CEO is told about available job. CEO says he is not interested.   Brief

Tuesday (11.5 hours)

Activities and Episodes   **Time Spent**

1. CEO informs another hospital CEO about the search for his successor. Later this is discussed with the board chairman and the VP for human services. (I am asked not to attend this meeting.)   Long

2. CEO of another hospital advises of a mutual friend who is an inpatient and who would like to be visited.   Brief

3. CEO discusses with full-time physician the physician's visiting affiliated hospitals to discuss managed care. Later, CEO calls chief of service to clear the visits.   Intermediate

4. CEO is informed by associate administrator of community meeting about relocation plan related to sale of property and of related local politics.   Brief

5. CEO is informed about a second state-investigated patient complaint which must be followed up on.   Brief

6. CEO is informed by chief engineer and COO that trustee-donated suite can be visited; CEO tours the suite.   Intermediate

7. CEO is informed by COO that a VIP patient is much better today.   Brief

8. CEO asks COO whether someone would be interested in a job he received a letter about.   Brief

9. CEO is called by lawyer regarding progress in preparing for malpractice case. Calls second lawyer twice in regard to handling of the case.   Brief

10. Lobbyist calls about visit to senator concerning funding for graduate education.   Brief

11. Lobbyist's call also concerns land preservation law which is blocking hospital property development.   Brief

12. CEO meets with director of a chaplaincy organization who is requesting space and money for ongoing program.   Intermediate

13. Trustee calls about item for discussion at board meeting. Associate administrator calls twice about removing an item from the agenda.   Brief

14. CFO calls regarding who will attend another meeting.   Brief

15. CEO meets with two trustees and three administrators about cleanliness of the hospital.   Long

16. They also discuss food services.   Intermediate

17. CEO is informed by assistant administrator of VIP's health status and satisfaction with room.   Brief

18. Assistant administrator asks whether CEO can meet with management students.   Brief

19. CEO attends meeting across town of local hospital association.   Very Long

Wednesday (11.5 hours)

Activities and Episodes	Time Spent
1. CEO meets with department chairman regarding the search for the CEO's successor.	Brief
2. CEO discusses lobbying on federal tax legislation with associate administrator and with lawyer.	Brief
3. Associate administrator informs CEO of progress with historic preservation and land development; CEO discusses with board chairman and with lawyer.	Brief
4. CEO discusses JCAH letter regarding bylaws' responsibility for quality assurance, to be on agenda at board meeting.	Brief
5. Assistant administrator informs CEO of health status of a VIP patient.	Brief
6. Assistant administrator asks about her place on the medical executive committee agenda.	Brief
7. Community relations officer asks CEO to tour apartments relative to relocation plan and to discuss local politics. CEO tours apartments to which tenants will be relocated; attends community meeting about relocation and discusses with CFO what happened after he left the meeting.	Long
8. CEO meets with board chairman, medical school dean, and director of development about interinstitutional research and related fund raising.	Long
9. Board chairman informs CEO of meeting on technological progress in certain medical specialties.	Brief
10. Secretary asks CEO for medical advice for a patient. CEO talks to the patient, calls physician, and dictates note to physician.	Brief
11. Progress report on executive registry for patient care in other cities is discussed at staff meeting of about ten administrators.	Brief
12. At meeting, CEO tells CFO to report to board results of monitoring the impact of DRGs.	Brief
13. At meeting, VP for human resources informs staff of managerial merit increase plan.	Brief
14. At meeting, associate administrator reports to staff on construction progress.	Brief

15. At meeting, COO reports to staff on plan to close   Brief
    patient floors if occupancy declines.

16. At meeting, COO discusses with staff new report   Brief
    on one-day stays.

17. At meeting, VP for human resources requests state-   Brief
    ments of objectives.

18. At meeting, CEO requests information on who is   Brief
    attending local interinstitutional meeting.

19. At meeting, CEO shares his views of the hospital's   Brief
    proposed approach to managed care.

20. Assistant administrator tells CEO of mistakes in   Brief
    procedures manual.

21. CEO discusses three times with attorney a letter   Brief
    being written to a public official regarding a mal-
    practice case.

22. CEO discusses with in-house attorney inclusion of   Brief
    managed care on board meeting agenda.

23. CEO discusses twice with associate administrator   Brief
    who will attend a meeting in Washington.

24. CEO asks associate administrator whether a meet-   Brief
    ing took place regarding space for staff residence.

25. CEO meets with three clinical chairmen and COO   Brief
    about medical board meeting agenda.

26. Staff appointments discussed at medical board ex-   Brief
    ecutive committee of about 20 physicians.

27. Ambulatory surgery guidelines discussed at meeting.   Brief

28. Shared radiation therapy with another hospital dis-   Brief
    cussed. (I am asked to leave the meeting for reasons
    of confidentiality.) COO informs CEO of what hap-
    pened after CEO left meeting.

29. CEO discusses with a full-time physician affiliations   Brief
    program with other hospitals.

30. CEO is driven to meet with PR consultant regarding   Long
    preparation for hearing on malpractice case. (I am
    asked not to attend.) CEO informs COO of meeting.

31. Physician asks CEO in hall what the hospital is   Brief
    doing about HMOs.

32. CEO suggests to other hospital CEO that CEO of   Brief
    third hospital should attend monthly meeting of
    hospital administrators.

33. Trustee calls CEO about board procedure for approving capital equipment requests. — Brief
34. CEO reviews with COO the hospitals already affiliated with Washington Medical Center. — Brief
35. CEO visits inpatient who is VIP. — Brief
36. CEO visits inpatient who is an employee. — Brief
37. CEO discusses with assistant administrator the do-not-resuscitate memo and its communication to the house staff. — Brief

Larry Martin, CEO of Van Buren Hospital

Monday (8 hours)

Activities and Episodes	Time Spent
1. CEO informs COO of process of disengagement from contract with a second hospital for shared OB-GYN services. CEO is informed by cochiefs of OB-GYN department that they intend to proceed with disengagement. Discusses this with CEO of a third hospital.	Long
2. CEO asks CEO of third hospital whether anyone else should attend a merger meeting; schedules merger talks. CEO meets with CEO of third hospital and with consultants regarding possible merger or consolidation of services. CEO informs board chairman of merger talks. CEO informs COO and another senior administrator of merger talks.	Long
3. CEO supplies COO with letter decertifying six beds.	Brief
4. Pediatrician requests meeting with CEO about joint hospital-M.D. ventures.	Brief
5. CEO schedules meeting with the administrator of another hospital after a medical school consortium meeting.	Brief
6. CEO discusses managed care at meeting with CEO of third hospital and with consultants.	Brief
7. CEO discusses Van Buren Hospital's for-profit company with CEO of third hospital.	Brief
8. CEO calls hospital attorney regarding purchase of apartment owned by the hospital for the CEO.	Brief

9. CEO is informed of possible refusal by board member to chair a dinner dance (conflict of interest). — Brief

10. CEO decides that senior administrator, rather than the CEO, should welcome visitors to alcoholism event. — Brief

11. CEO is informed that a government official wants to talk about continuation of a grant and additional funding for expanded operations. — Brief

Tuesday (8.2 hours)

Activities and Episodes	Time Spent
1. COO informs CEO of financial arrangements with returning chief of service. COO later tells CEO that this chief met with the CEO of the second hospital and that Van Buren CEO should call the CEO of the second hospital.	Intermediate
2. CEO asks COO why rehabilitation census is not higher.	Brief
3. CEO discusses with COO patient origins, which are relevant to merger discussions with third hospital. CEO talks with CEO of third hospital, then tells COO of discussion. Drives to third hospital to discuss with its CEO and two members of each hospital's board the possible merger; dinner followed.	Very Long
4. CEO meets with five other administrative staff to discuss for-profit subsidiary: nurse registry rates, lab contract, and malpractice insurance for technicians.	Long
5. Physician asks CEO how to respond to IPA being formed by the medical staff.	Intermediate
6. Associate administrator (AA1) asks about use of board room for site visit.	Brief
7. Another associate administrator (AA2) shares information about possible contract to manage housing complex.	Brief
8. AA1 discusses possible contract with social maintenance organization for family practice care.	Brief
9. AA2 asks about rental charge for use of hospital space.	Brief
10. COO discusses possible problem in shared radiation therapy services with second hospital.	Brief

11. CEO discusses with wife insurance on hospital-purchased co-op apartment. Earlier, CEO deals with writing check for this.	Brief
12. CEO and AA2 meet with two staff of an HMO to discuss possible HMO linkages with the hospital.	Long

Wednesday (10.75 hours)

Activities and Episodes	Time Spent
1. CEO and AA2 discuss HMO meeting of yesterday.	Brief
2. AA2 reports on medical staff IPA meeting of last night.	Brief
3. COO reports that returning chief wants commitment on bottom-line financials before return. Later, CEO reviews allocation of functions between returning and existing chief. CEO calls CEO of second hospital about merger phase-out.	Intermediate
4. CEO reviews merger meeting of last night with AA2 and COO, then with chief of service, then with AA1. CEO discusses composition of merger steering committee.	Brief
5. CEO calls CEO of a fourth hospital about getting together at a meeting in Washington.	Brief
6. AA2 asks CEO whether CEO wishes to meet with another HMO.	Brief
7. CEO discusses with AA1 the managing of an additional satellite health center.	Brief
8. CEO discusses with VP for personnel the labor negotiations with hospital nurses.	Brief
9. CEO greets former employee now working on a grant proposal.	Brief
10. CEO calls lawyer on co-op lease.	Brief
11. CEO drives to medical school advisory council meeting, where legislation affecting flexibility in budgeting and accreditation visits are discussed.	Long

Ted Grover, CEO of Cleveland Hospital

Monday (12.25 hours)

Activities and Episodes	Time Spent
1. CEO is informed by COO of phone threat to VP of human resources.	Brief

2. CEO is informed by COO that applicant has ac-   Brief
   cepted offer as new chief of genetics.

3. CEO is informed by COO of office space mix-up   Brief
   involving physician whom the hospital is attempting
   to fire.

4. CEO is informed by clinical chief of perceived in-   Brief
   effective behavior of another clinical chief.

5. After being informed by COO of preparations   Brief
   underway for the state health department inspec-
   tion survey, CEO responds that he will meet state
   surveyors.

6. CEO requests information from COO concerning   Brief
   drop in census.

7. CEO informs COO about the progress in planning   Brief
   hospital budget reductions.

8. CEO informs COO regarding implementation of   Brief
   changes in the hospital's fringe benefit plan.

9. CEO informs COO about MRI lease.   Brief

10. CEO informs COO about progress on a second site   Brief
    construction budget.

11. CEO is informed by COO about cost and produc-   Brief
    tivity information that may be available for each
    hospital cost center.

12. CEO tells COO about continuation of captive mal-   Brief
    practice insurance company involving other hospi-
    tals as well.

13. CEO informs COO of arrangements for delayed   Brief
    payments to pension fund.

14. CEO informs COO that he will review executive   Brief
    committee meeting later with CFO.

15. CEO discusses merger with another hospital CEO   Very Long
    and consultants. All parties request further infor-
    mation from each other.

16. CEO tells CFO about progress in rate adjustment   Brief
    by the state. CEO then asks CFO to get information
    about obtaining increased state reimbursement.

17. In response to information about a donation to the   Brief
    second site, the CEO requests that the COO of that
    site channel the donation through the hospital de-
    velopment program.

18. CEO is informed by the COO about awards cere-   Brief
    mony at second site.
19. After being informed about proposed state malprac- Brief
    tice insurance rates and legislation, CEO responds
    to trade association secretary that he can't attend
    a meeting.
20. CEO agrees to use of his name to sponsor charitable Brief
    luncheon for medical disease organization.
21. CEO tells secretary that he cannot attend a medical Brief
    school consortium meeting.
22. After being informed of options in reorganizing state Brief
    payment for uncompensated care, CEO tells CEO
    of another hospital his preference.
23. CEO is told by VP of medical affairs about the   Brief
    planned dismissal of a physician.
24. CEO is informed by assistant administrator of im-   Brief
    plementation of hospital's quality assurance
    program.

Tuesday (9.5 hours)

Activities and Episodes	Time Spent
1. CEO discusses complaint about clinical chief with the president of the medical staff.	Brief
2. Administrative assistant reports on the census. Chief of surgery calls, saying census is up. CEO reports this to board chairman.	Brief
3. Trustee shows up for meeting scheduled for tomorrow.	Brief
4. CEO discusses with assistant administrator eliminating hospital funding of M.D. fellows.	Brief
5. CEO discusses with trustee understanding of prior agreements with already merged hospital.	Brief
6. CEO discusses with board chairman the hiring of an M.D.	Brief
7. CEO discusses budget reduction plan, to be on board meeting agenda, with assistant administrator.	Brief
8. CEO discusses the construction program and a problem with minority hiring, also on the board's agenda. Later, CEO meets with five administrators to review progress on the above and contingency plans if revenue targets are not met.	Brief

9. CEO discusses hospital diversification with assis-   Brief
   tant administrator. CEO later meets with five administrators to review specific diversification
   projects.

10. CEO discusses malpractice insurance overpayment   Brief
    with CFO.

11. CEO discusses with CFO his performance evalua-   Intermediate
    tion. (I am asked not to be present.) Later, CEO
    discusses this with board chairman.

12. CEO discusses malpractice rates with CFO.   Brief

13. CEO discusses a malpractice case with CFO.   Brief

14. CEO discusses state rate reimbursement with CFO.   Brief
    CEO discusses this later with board chairman.

15. CEO reviews consultant's report on merger with   Brief
    other hospital; asks CFO to respond to questions
    about the merger.

16. CEO reviews board resolutions on amendments to   Brief
    the hospital pension plan. CEO discusses this later
    with board chairman.

17. CEO reviews organization and structure of captive   Brief
    malpractice insurance company. Later, CEO dis-
    cusses reimbursement of consultant to this company.

18. Chief of surgery calls CEO regarding inflation clause   Brief
    in his contract.

19. CEO meets with medical affairs coordinator to dis-   Brief
    cuss her dismissal, then meets with COO and assis-
    tant administrator regarding it. CEO is asked to
    sign goodbye card; later discusses dismissal with
    board chairman.

20. CEO discusses quality assurance filing system with   Brief
    assistant administrator.

21. CEO calls board chairman in regard to board meet-   Brief
    ing agenda. CEO reviews this with COO as well.
    CEO meets with board chairman about agenda.

22. CEO calls VP of human resources regarding arbi-   Brief
    tration over pension payments. CEO mentions this
    later at meeting with three administrators.

23. CEO meets with three other administrators   Long
    about organizing services relating to disability
    examinations.

24. CEO discusses organization and marketing of pri-   Intermediate
    mary care unit with these three administrators. CEO
    later tells board chairman this unit is losing money.

25. Chairman discusses annual trustee seminar with   Brief
    CEO. CEO discusses this later with development
    officer.

26. Chairman relates to CEO patient complaint about   Brief
    ER service.

27. CEO reports to board chairman on date of JCAH   Brief
    survey.

28. CEO reports to board chairman on state reimburse-   Brief
    ment in light of recent court decisions.

29. Board chairman asks CEO about no-smoking policy.   Brief

30. CEO reviews results of a recent development fund-   Brief
    raising event.

31. CEO mentions problems in future of medical school   Brief
    affiliations program.

32. Board chairman asks about new medical staff   Brief
    appointments.

33. CEO discusses with chairman of board attendance   Brief
    at an awards ceremony.

34. CEO calls director of development regarding re-   Brief
    sponsibility for organizing hospital fund-raising
    event.

35. CEO reviews capital budgeting process with devel-   Brief
    opment officer.

36. CEO discusses changes in bylaws with assistant   Brief
    administrator.

Wednesday (10.5 hours)

Activities and Episodes   **Time Spent**

1. Attorney calls CEO about state malpractice legis-   Intermediate
   lation. CEO discusses this later with VP of medical
   affairs and subsequently with others regarding malpractice rate increase.

2. CEO attends meeting of operations and planning   Brief
   committee, with 11 others, about quality assurance
   in relation to state regulation and JCAH survey.

3. At meeting, CEO discusses rate reimbursement.   Brief
   Later, CFO reports on progress after discussion with
   rate regulator. Still later, CEO tells CFO of his discussion with regulator.

4. At meeting, assistant administrator reviews hospital   Intermediate
   construction program.

5. At meeting, assistant administrator reviews diver-   Brief
   sification program.

6. At meeting, COO reviews classifications system for   Brief
   emergency medical care.

7. CEO presents research proposal sent by trustee to   Brief
   VP of medical affairs.

8. CEO discusses the recent termination with VP of   Intermediate
   medical affairs. Later, CEO looks at gift, gives
   speech at goodbye party, and asks secretary how
   the goodbye party went after he left.

9. CEO discusses need for women's health program   Brief
   with VP of medical affairs; later tells COO to convene meeting on this. COO later suggests reviewing
   others' women's health programs.

10. VP of medical affairs urges CEO to take complaint   Brief
    about clinical chief seriously.

11. Meeting with three administrators on implementa-   Brief
    tion of fringe benefits revisions.

12. CEO discusses with CFO letter about arbitration.   Brief

13. CEO asks CFO for comments on consultants' re-   Brief
    port on merger.

14. Conference call, with three other persons, to dis-   Long
    cuss local hospital association's position on state
    reimbursement.

15. CEO reviews with development officer CEO's pres-   Brief
    entation of grant program results to granting agency.

16. CEO reviews development priorities and donations   Intermediate
    process with development officer.

17. CEO reviews with development officer marketing   Brief
    programs for health center, women's health, and
    merged hospital.

18. Lawyer calls CEO about strategy for malpractice   Brief
    case meeting. CEO calls assistant administrator
    about this. Later CEO discusses this with VP of
    medical affairs.

19. CEO discusses trustee seminar with development officer.   Brief

20. CFO calls about report of auditor regarding parking garage. CEO meets with CFO and auditor about other problems in parking charges not collected. CEO dictates memo on policy and collection of fees. Later, CEO discusses this with assistant administrator.   Long

21. CEO asks development officer about recommendations for salary increases for his staff.   Brief

22. CEO comments that surgeon doesn't want to treat an AIDS patient with an appendix problem.   Brief

23. CEO meets with VP of medical affairs and COO and with clinical chief about whom there are complaints. They discuss complaints, staffing, and strategy. Later, CEO discusses the situation with VP of medical affairs.   Long

24. Chairman of board calls, saying that M.D. complained about the growing number of hospital administrators.   Brief

25. Assistant administrator discusses ending hospital payment for medical resident from another hospital.   Brief

Sam Woodrow, CEO of Wilson HMO

Monday (10.5 hours)

Activities and Episodes	Time Spent
1. CEO exchanges information about options regarding mergers and acquisitions at meeting with five other administrators. Later, CEO requests administrative assistant to touch base with others before the next meeting, to rank options.	Long
2. CEO carries out performance appraisal of a manager. (I am asked not to be present.)	Long
3. CEO makes follow-up call to job applicant.	Intermediate
4. CEO responds to medical group director's request for expansion of facilities.	Long
5. CEO informs medical group director of the desirability of one, rather than many, medical groups.	Brief

6. CEO is informed by medical group director of physicians' perceptions of an owned hospital.   Brief

7. CEO responds to request to discuss performance appraisals of other managers with COO tomorrow.   Brief

8. CEO responds to request for a decision regarding another CEO's application for membership in HMO trade organization.   Brief

9. CEO tells trade association official about grant request to a foundation.   Brief

10. CEO is informed at large annual lab meeting about joint laboratory operations.   Long

11. CEO responds to CFO's request for a decision about payment level to physicians in a new PPO.   Brief

12. CEO is informed by CFO of auditor's letter relating to rate payment by city government. Later, at managers' meeting, is informed of new performance clause in its contracts.   Brief

13. CEO is informed by PR officer of press conference on hospital affiliation; PR officer later informs the 11 persons at managers' meeting.   Intermediate

14. CEO determines with COO that a particular benefit is the type of political activity that Wilson cannot purchase tickets for.   Brief

15. CEO responds to PR officer's request concerning wording of memo about changed organizational responsibility for publications.   Brief

16. CEO responds to PR officer's request concerning press release relating to former board chairman.   Brief

17. CEO is informed by PR officer of press conference on second HMO site; PR officer later informs at managers' meeting.   Brief

18. At managers' meeting, CEO is informed by CFO about competitive PPO product.   Brief

19. At meeting, CEO discusses new budget sent to the state insurance department.   Brief

20. At meeting, CEO is told by attorney of implementation of policy requiring specialists to have passed specialty boards.   Brief

21. At meeting, CEO is told by staff that fire damage to ambulatory center has been repaired.   Brief

22. At meeting, CEO is informed of the progress of the capital facilities construction program.   Brief

23. At meeting, CEO is told about implementation of new telephone service system.   Brief

24. At meeting, CEO is informed of possible offer of HMO plan to another union.   Brief

25. At meeting, CEO is informed of rates and performances of new HMO competitors.   Brief

26. At meeting, CEO is informed about negotiating with a new advertising firm concerning fall advertising campaign.   Brief

27. At meeting, CEO is informed of changes in city personnel which may affect Wilson HMO.   Brief

28. At meeting, CEO is informed of progress in responding to consumer complaints.   Brief

29. At meeting, CEO is told of implementation date of new PPO.   Brief

30. CEO discusses with others performance of managers in certain departments. (I was not present.)   Long

Tuesday (9.25 hours)

Activities and Episodes	Time Spent
1. CEO calls Wilson medical director about serving on national committee on technology assessment.	Intermediate
2. CEO reviews with associate administrator speech to be presented at press conference to celebrate hospital affiliation. CEO gives remarks at affiliated hospital; about 100 people attend. Later, CEO reviews press release with administrative assistant. Medical group director calls CEO with positive feedback.	Long
3. CEO reviews planning and corporate development budget with associate administrator.	Brief
4. CEO discusses corporate reorganization with associate administrator.	Intermediate
5. CEO discusses performance appraisal of manager with associate administrator.	Brief
6. CEO discusses new manager in the medical department with associate administrator.	Brief

7. CFO tells CEO they need board members to attend   Intermediate
   Wilson Hospital survey visit. CEO mentions survey
   to hospital attending physicians at hospital press
   conference lunch. CEO discusses by phone with
   Wilson Hospital's administrator how the survey is
   going. Later, he reviews this discussion with COO.
   COO and associate administrator can't attend survey meeting because of meeting with city politician.

8. In car, CEO discusses Wilson Hospital facilities with   Brief
   CFO.

9. In car, CEO discusses merger of medical groups   Brief
   with CFO.

10. In car, CEO discusses appointment access and hours   Brief
    of operation of medical groups with CFO.

11. In car, CEO discusses introduction of new PPO   Brief
    product with CFO. Later, CFO discusses finalizing
    of claims administrations agreement for the PPO.

12. In car, CEO discusses refinancing of lab services   Brief
    with CFO.

13. In car, CEO discusses meeting with president of   Brief
    claims administration organization with CFO.

14. In car, CEO discusses with CFO recruitment of COO   Long
    for Wilson subsidiary. Discusses later with associ-
    ate administrator last interview with candidate and
    timing of hire relative to scheduled press conference
    for the subsidiary; discusses also the organizational
    relationship of subsidiary to main unit. Discusses
    twice with the medical director of the subsidiary
    the scheduling of the subsidiary board meeting.
    Discusses whether he should attend press confer-
    ence (with PR officer). CEO discusses hiring recruit
    with the administrator of the subsidiary. Later, CEO
    discusses recruiting strategy with COO.

15. CEO tells Wilson attorney that the medical group   Brief
    director should attend the subsidiary board meeting.

16. CEO talks with consumer representatives at lunch-   Brief
    eon about correspondence from retirees.

17. At luncheon, CEO talks with medical school dean   Brief
    and later with hospital CFO about medical school
    teaching at Wilson.

18. At luncheon, attending physicians and staff inquire   Brief
    of CEO about rate increase.

19. At luncheon, CEO discusses HMO benefits for hos-   Brief
    pital employees with Wilson hospital administrator.
20. CEO arranges meeting with another medical group   Brief
    director about his budget.
21. CEO discusses press conference about subsidiary   Brief
    with PR director.
22. On phone, CEO answers question about an excep-   Brief
    tion to the enrollment policy in Wilson HMO.
23. CEO instructs administrative assistant to fill out na- Brief
    tional HMO survey form.
24. CEO discusses twice with administrative assistant   Brief
    the reorganization of the communications function.
25. Consultant calls CEO to help in obtaining funding   Intermediate
    for a research project.
26. COO asks CEO about policy regarding a different   Brief
    type of fund-raising event.
27. CEO discusses with administrative assistant meet-   Brief
    ing about merger with another HMO and the need
    for another planning meeting regarding merger op-
    tions. CEO discusses purchase of an HMO in an-
    other state.
28. Administrative assistant discusses affirmative action   Brief
    meeting and hiring of minority kids for the summer.
29. CEO calls board member about planning and meet-   Brief
    ing to plan reorganization of HMO malpractice
    insurance.
30. Associate administrator reviews strategy options   Brief
    discussed on Monday with CFO and how these
    should be organized and ranked.
31. CEO leaves to attend function for governor.   Brief

Wednesday (10.0 hours)

Activities and Episodes   **Time Spent**
1. CFO reviews proposals from three consultants re-   Brief
   garding handling of investments; this is discussed
   at executive board meeting.
2. CEO calls Wilson hospital administrator about ac-   Brief
   creditation survey meeting.

3. CFO asks at meeting of CEO and two other admin-   Intermediate
    istrators about review of the capital budget. Capital
    budget is discussed at Wilson executive board
    meeting.

4. At salary review meeting, CEO discusses with three   Long
    other administrators exceptional raises for staff.

5. Attorney asks CEO for letter of support for bill pro-   Brief
    posed in state legislature regarding city health de-
    partment. They discuss it again later. Still later, CEO
    reviews the attorney's letter.

6. CEO reviews with CFO, in the car on the way to   Brief
    the hospital for accreditation survey meeting, their
    perceptions of the hospital—its facilities, morale,
    and staffing.

7. CEO and CFO review strategy relative to meeting   Brief
    with claims intermediary.

8. They discuss refinancing the lab building; this is   Brief
    discussed later at executive board meeting.

9. They discuss a medical group director's request for   Brief
    additional center space.

10. CEO attends meeting with accreditors and listens   Long
    to the report.

11. On car ride back, attorney speaks to CEO regarding   Brief
    letter of support for federal tax legislation.

12. CFO instructs attorney to have HMO membership   Brief
    applications ready for new board members and to
    process separately.

13. CEO discusses with administrative assistant request   Brief
    from congressman about paying a patient's claim.

14. CEO discusses personnel matter with COO. (I am   Intermediate
    asked not to be present.)

15. CEO discusses malpractice case with COO. (I am   Brief
    asked not to be present.)

16. CFO indicates to CEO that capital budget does not   Brief
    include equipment.

17. CEO reviews meeting schedules and dates with   Brief
    secretary.

18. CEO reviews who will attend meeting with   Brief
    congressman.

19. CEO attends with board members, staff, and con-   Long
sultants an audit committee meeting to review consultant report.

20. CEO attends executive board meeting, where he   Brief
discusses financing of CT scanner.

21. CEO discusses operating budget at executive board   Intermediate
meeting.

22. CEO discusses HMO benefit for mental health serv-   Brief
ices staff.

Activities Related to One Managerial Episode that Spanned Three Days

Tim George, Managed Care

Monday

1. CEO from another academic health center calls and says that his hospital will not be part of an HMO's managed care plan.

2. CEO discusses managed care with an M.D. job applicant interested in working part time in administration.

3. CEO discusses with top planner the forming of a physician organization for managed care, informing the board, and developing affiliations with other hospitals.

4. CEO reads consultant's report on the strategy the hospital should follow in regard to managed care.

5. CEO arranges meeting for Tuesday with physician who is responsible for developing hospital affiliations.

Tuesday

6. CEO discusses strategy for developing affiliations with responsible physician; CEO undertakes to clear the additional time involved with the physician's clinical chief.

7. CEO speaks to the clinical chief about what the physician will be doing in regard to affiliations.

Wednesday

8. CEO discusses with managerial staff the dimensions of managed care, including organizational questions, enrollment of physicians, equity for development and sales, hospital affiliations, and marketing.

9. CEO discusses with associate clinical chairman the participation of a physician in managing the affiliation program.
10. CEO is asked by an attending physician what the hospital's position on managed care is. CEO responds that hospital is exploring it.
11. CEO and COO go over those hospitals with which Washington Medical Center currently has affiliations.

Larry Martin, Shared OB-GYN Services

Monday

1. CEO reviews the situation with his COO. He wants to reconfirm that Dr. B, a codirector of OB-GYN, will return to Van Buren Hospital after the agreement for shared services is terminated. This was agreed to by both parties if merger talks failed.
2. CEO meets with the codirectors of OB-GYN and the COO. CEO summarizes his position, and the codirectors agree with the summary. CEO says he will attempt to satisfy Dr. B professionally and financially and wants to know when he can return to Van Buren Hospital. Dr. B says whenever it is agreeable to the two CEOs. CEO concludes by saying he wants to strengthen Van Buren's clinical service.
3. CEO tells the CEO of a third hospital, with whom he is conducting merger talks, about the second hospital's offer to hire Dr. B and that Dr. B will be returning to Van Buren Hospital.

Tuesday

4. CEO meets with COO, who says that the two codirectors are satisfied with the financial package, which will be more costly, and with who should be in charge of what between them.
5. CEO meets with COO, who says Dr. B called. Dr. B told the medical director of the second hospital about his decision and said that CEO Martin would be calling the second hospital's CEO. Dr. B will meet with the medical director of the second hospital on Thursday. CEO says that now this is Dr. B's decision. COO says to the CEO, I didn't want to hear what their hospital had to offer; I told Dr. B that Van Buren Hospital would be fair.

Wednesday

6. CEO meets with COO, who says the codirectors want a bottom-line commitment before Dr. B leaves the second hospital. Dr. B wants the same money he's currently earning without taking the money from his codirector, Dr. C. CEO says that, for the money, Dr. B can build

a department with young obstetricians and Van Buren will also get a director of medical education. This gives the hospital some of Dr. C's time as merger talks proceed. CEO asks the COO to write down the quid pro quos for all parties.

7. Dr. B drops by, and the CEO reviews merger talks with him. Dr. B doesn't want Dr. C to step down prematurely. He says that the timing has to be resolved. The CEO says that Dr. B should concentrate on what has to be done to make the service relevant in the marketplace. He will continue as director of medical education. The CEO will ask Dr. C to represent the clinical directors in merger talks.

8. CEO calls the CEO of the second hospital about terminating the shared service agreement. He says that Dr. B indicates he wants to return home to Van Buren Hospital. Does the other CEO have any thoughts on the matter? CEO says that once someone has decided to leave, their staying will be ineffective, so the quicker the better.

Ted Grover, Complaints About a Chief of Service

Monday

1. The COO informs the CEO that a clinical chief received a call from the president of the medical board indicating that they must get rid of a new chief, Dr. L, who is a "menace." An attending physician, Dr. P, wants to know if Dr. L's decision to dismiss him will be reversed. Another clinical chief has suggested open discussion. The CEO reviews Dr. L's plan concerning phase-out of Dr. P. The CEO says that the changes Dr. L wants to make are appropriate, but not the way he's doing it.

Tuesday

2. The president of the medical board calls the CEO about a social engagement, and the CEO asks him, How are things with Dr. L's service?

Wednesday

3. The vice-president of medical affairs, in a meeting about diversification, tells the CEO, Take the Dr. L thing seriously: they're building it up!

4. The CEO meets with Dr. L, the COO, and the vice-president of medical affairs. The CEO says:

> This is a follow-up of other meetings concerning your service. We support you in what has to be done. Some people complain about the speed and the manner of those charges, implying insensitivity on your part.

Political groups are forming that can create problems for you and us. Our compromise included a phase-out of Dr. P. Three things have happened: (1) the rumor mill has ground out venom, creating trouble between full-time and voluntary staff; (2) the people involved have developed anxiety and insecurity, wondering if they will be targets; and (3) an official appeal has been made to the professional staff by persons in the department, and the organized medical staff has requested a statement of policy by the hospital indicating that something must be done.

Dr. L complains about members of his department who were working elsewhere while working at Cleveland Hospital, overpaying of certain physicians, poor training of residents, and how he has tried to work things out about phasing out Dr. P.

The vice-president of medical affairs says that his interest is to preserve the integrity of the department—we're not trying to reverse decisions, the problem is how things are done.

The CEO says that they must do something to indicate responsiveness to what people perceive, says that Dr. P should be retired at age 72, and asks how Dr. L intends to deal with others in the department whom he wishes to remove. The CEO suggests that they be dismissed, that they be paid well, that the president of the medical staff be informed, and that perhaps a committee be formed for better communications. The CEO concludes by stating that they must demonstrate sensitivity regarding Dr. P. The CEO will tell the president of the medical staff what is planned, and they will all meet with the president of the medical board.

Sam Woodrow, Recruitment of a Chief Operating Officer for a Wilson Subsidiary

Monday

1. CEO responds to job applicant on the phone that he is not among the final two or three candidates for the position but that he should come back for another interview if he is interested in any of the new management opportunities that will be opening up.
2. CEO tells his secretary when the preferred applicant will visit for an interview, indicates whom the applicant should meet with and for how long, and asks her to make hotel reservations.

Tuesday

3. CEO discusses the leading candidate for the position with the CFO in a cab ride to an affiliated hospital, where they are holding a joint press conference.

4. CEO meets with the associate administrator. They discuss the leading candidate: his strengths and his weaknesses, how he will fit with the current administrator and medical director, and how the position will relate to management staff at Wilson HMO headquarters. The CEO discusses what the new person's priorities should be, whether he thinks the candidate will accept, changes that may have to be made in the satellite governing board, and whether, if the applicant accepts, an announcement should be made at next week's press conference, if that can be arranged. After calling to begin the process of satellite board approval, the CEO changes his mind. He says he doesn't want to rush their regular executive board meeting. The new man should be introduced to physicians, and he may want time to announce it to his own organization.

5. The CEO calls the administrator of the subsidiary and asks whether he wants to talk with the CEO alone or to wait until a final decision is made concerning a new COO. The CEO states, I'm willing to talk to you about your concerns, about how you will relate to a new COO. The CEO tells the administrator not to worry, that he is held in high esteem by people at headquarters, including the CEO.

Part Three

Interpretation and Implications

*Administrators in this town play not to lose—
they don't play to win. They spend more time
covering their rear and not being exposed, to
minimize criticism. The problem with most of
these places is they are hand-to-mouth
operations, and the manager's orientation is to
cash flow. Cash management has been
elevated to a high art form, which lessens your
creativity in other areas.*

—Hospital lobbyist, Spring 1986

7.

Crosscutting Themes

I can reach no conclusions about "the effective manager" in large health care organizations because the interview data are not summable. What made for an effective manager in one set of circumstances was not the same as in another, even though the four CEOs headed large health care organizations in the same city. Based on the data, however, I have developed some themes that appear to be common to effective management in large health care organizations: (1) the importance of periodically setting CEO and trustee expectations regarding CEO performance, (2) the lack of transferability of CEOs across large health organizations, (3) the importance of visible results as related to CEO choice in managing work, and (4) the impact of increasing size and complexity of health organizations upon the structure and function of the executive office.

Setting CEO and Trustee Expectations Regarding CEO Performance

Large health care organizations are difficult to manage effectively because of differing opinions on mission and on the contribution of management to organizational effectiveness. Health care organizations are political organizations. As the chief financial officer at Wilson HMO observes:

> Health care is a very regulated industry—and health organizations function in a very political environment. . . . Issues are resolved more slowly, and we get involved with the political structure. . . . Your production is your doctors, so you have to find ways to work with physicians who are independent and don't have a real sense of what the consumer wants.

Health care organizations may be more constrained in responding to changing business conditions. As a nursing administrator at Van Buren Hospital remarks:

> In a business it's more for yourself. A not-for-profit institution is under so much regulation, and more uncertainty as to income, that you can't just raise your prices. It's more difficult, you don't get paid more for doing better. We've got to be more cost-conscious.

Regarding disagreement on organizational objectives in large health care organizations, the board chairman of Cleveland Hospital contrasts health care with business organizations:

> It's a little more difficult than in business, working together for the benefit of the hospital. Eastern Airlines has one aim, and you don't have to worry about two or three groups. There lies the seed of real problems.

And health services managers have less power as managers. As a clinical chief at Washington Medical Center observes:

> The hospital administrator's job depends on the whims of the practicing staff, and the administrator knows that.

At Washington Medical Center, the board and CEO Tim George are moving to what George terms "a more quantitative assessment [of objectives], one based on what we have projected." George has difficulty, however, in setting his own expectations regarding CEO performance:

> I aggregate administrators' goal statements and include things that I think are particularly important. I found that my objectives were included in others', and I wanted to give them credit.

The four CEOs are not evaluated in terms of their contribution to organizational effectiveness, nor is "organizational effectiveness" specified. Regarding his evaluation at Wilson HMO, CEO Sam Woodrow says:

> Evaluation of my performance occurs at two levels. On an ongoing basis, I will know very quickly if the board has lost confidence in me. Conversely, if the board continues to support my proposals as they have, this becomes in essence my review. I do, however, have an annual review with the chairman of the board. This tends to be very results-oriented. I am evaluated on the leadership I have provided. This is a positive experience because it is objective.

"Results-oriented" is not determined, however, on the basis of preset, mutually agreed-upon, measurable objectives. Although expectations are not explicitly set and CEO performance is not evaluated relative to them in the organizations studied, some implicit expectations were set during the hiring process of each CEO. In two of the four organizations studied, expectations are also set implicitly during long-range planning processes among managers, trustees, and medical staff.

CEO George states that when he was first hired:

> The assumption was that the hospital would run modest deficits—it always had because of the free care it provides. They hoped the financial situation would improve but not at the expense of the mission of the hospital.

The trustees appear to be telling George that they want him to improve the financial situation of the hospital but not at the expense of its mission. (Implicitly, George is not seen as playing a leadership role in changing or specifying mission.)

Similarly, Larry Martin, CEO of Van Buren Hospital, says that when he was hired:

> I think the board hired me because they thought I was a good technician. I came from a nearby hospital which they thought highly of. They hoped [Van Buren] could be more like it, stronger and more stable. They got that. I spent the better part of my first two years here doing what I had learned how to do as a technician in order to improve the operation.

Martin's trustees appear to be telling him that his job is to improve the financial situation of the hospital so that it can be more like a neighboring hospital. (There is no mention of Martin's playing a leadership role with regard to mission or program, and Martin seems to have agreed to this, at least initially.)

With regard to a recent long-range planning process, George explains how the clinical chiefs shared with each other, for the first time in any formal way, their departmental objectives (presumably they developed and adapted these objectives relative to how they thought other chiefs were going to perceive them):

> The chiefs' objectives weren't out of line, they just didn't know the objectives of their colleagues. That's one of the things we have attempted to change by developing institutional objectives. We bring all the departments together and summarize plans and objectives for each other. . . . It was last done five years ago. We're updating plans now and will bring the chiefs together again.

This assembling of departmental objectives that are not related to a common financial framework is foreign to most large business firms.

The vice-president of medical affairs at Cleveland Hospital responds about a recent long-range planning process there:

We're ending a three-year plan and starting a new one. We have a retreat, invite experts to talk with us, and develop a modus operandi. Our last retreat was 18 months ago. The new plan (we brought in consultants) will have to do with capturing market share. How do we survive, cut costs, and provide quality care?

The vice-president uses the new business language of "market share" without specifying how or what agreement is reached with regard to how market share can be increased—and this in a hospital where many physicians who affect market share are not controlled by management and some even compete with the hospital in the provision of care.

Regarding the setting of organizational objectives, CEO Ted Grover of Cleveland Hospital speaks of satisfying

the clear objectives of a corporate mandate to provide accessible, high-quality human services to all persons, with public health programs and medical education as significant institutional responsibilities.

But how does the board or the medical staff at Cleveland Hospital know, for example, what are expected or acceptable levels of achievement regarding the provision of high-quality services? Or to what extent public health and medical education objectives are being met with regard to prenatal care, for example?

There are good reasons why neither organizational objectives nor CEO contribution to their attainment is being set in these large health care organizations. Among these reasons are (1) the lack of pressure to set objectives and (2) the cost, in conflict and time, of attempting to set them. I believe that it will be increasingly difficult, however, for large health care organizations to retain or gain market share in the future without setting expectations regarding organizational and CEO performance. Specifying organizational objectives is necessary for making and implementing decisions regarding scope of services at particular levels of cost and quality and for validating the CEO's role in making and implementing these decisions. Such specification is in the CEO's interest as well: it caps his or her risk by determining mutually and in advance what the objectives should be and what level of attainment can be expected under changing circumstances over which the CEO has little or no control. If the CEO attains the objectives, it is validation of his or her expected job performance, if not cause for raises in salary and bonuses.

Lack of Transferability of CEO Effectiveness across Large Health Organizations

Fiedler (1964, 1971) has emphasized that leadership characteristics vary with the situation; thus managers who are effective in one organi-

zation facing one set of circumstances may be ineffective in another organization facing different circumstances.

The four organizations studied vary with regard to mission, available
resources, political constituencies, organizational complexity, and turbu-
lence of environment. These differences, I believe, affect the work that
CEOs do and should do, as well as the roles they play and the functions
they perform.

On the circumstances that the CEO of Washington Medical Center
faces, George comments:

> The most important aspects of this job have to do with quality of patient care
> and enough . . . participation in the academic side to ensure that it is held
> up as well. . . . You must work with the chiefs to develop objectives that are
> consistent with institutional objectives but uniquely tailored to the needs of
> the departments. . . . It's a mistake to think that you will direct these people.
> You can influence them, but you don't tell them, This is what you're going
> to do.

Contrast this to Martin's observations on managing Van Buren
Hospital:

> I also leave behind the sense that the CEO is really the key: he sets the style,
> attitude, and spirit, signals whether it is a risk-taking place or not, defines
> institutional choices.

These two examples point up the differences between an effective
CEO in each organization. Martin is likely to involve himself more
thoroughly in fewer projects. If he participates less intensively in more
projects, which is how George must manage in order to be effective at
Washington Medical Center, he may manage less effectively. Conversely,
George might do poorly at Van Buren because his skills and experience
do not fit the organization's circumstances.

Because of disagreement about what large health care organizations
should do and how they can best produce their services, these organizations tend to require CEOs with well-developed political skills. As Sam
Woodrow, CEO of Wilson HMO, states,

> The CEO needs to balance several, at times competing, priorities in the Wil-
> son environment. It is necessary to take into consideration that our various
> constituents, the board, organized labor, our medical groups, and major ac-
> counts such as the city, may have differing interests on any given issue. I
> must seek consensus to move forward on major issues, and it often needs to
> be broad consensus. Moreover, the needs of our constituents must constantly
> be balanced with Wilson's needs in order to succeed in a highly competitive
> environment. This calls for strong political and negotiating skills. This also
> requires the CEO to be out front on issues—to be the consensus builder and
> not just sit back and wait for it to happen.

It is difficult for CEOs recruited from outside an organization to understand in sufficient detail the political networks required to implement agendas and for them to earn the trust of those whose support is necessary for significant change. As Woodrow observes about the effective CEO at Wilson HMO,

> You will be seriously hampered if you come in with specific goals and objectives but lack the management skills to adjust to new situations and new approaches and modifications. Power is fragmented in the Wilson environment; therefore, political skills are necessary to win support for objectives.

In accounting for the assumed effectiveness of the four CEOs studied, I am struck by their long tenures. This is in part why they were selected, but their tenures are even longer than I had stipulated. All four have been in their present positions for at least eight years. All four had been in their preceding positions for a similar period, either as CEO of a similar organization or as COO or clinical chief in the same or another organization. I believe tenure is related to perceived predictability of CEO behavior; this allows other leaders in the organization to focus on the work that must be done rather than on jockeying for position and worrying excessively about their job security and autonomy. As the chief operating officer of Cleveland Hospital observes about his superior, CEO Ted Grover:

> His tenure is a source of power. He was associate director for operations; his years of delivering to people have given him remarkable credibility, from department heads to clinicians.

Recruitment of a new CEO in large health care organizations may take many months, sometimes more than a year. Further, it is believed to be riskier than selecting a CEO in large business organizations because of the lack of agreement on technology and the conflicting goals in health care organizations. This is especially true when the new CEO is recruited from outside. The risk lies in eliciting the trust of a complex network of board members, medical staff leaders, and others whose support is required to implement a new agenda or to continue an existing one.

The need for a new agenda may be a key reason for recruiting from the outside. Choosing an insider may indicate an unwillingness or inability to agree upon changes that the organization needs in order to adapt successfully to a more competitive environment. This indicates to me the importance of setting mutual expectations and of planning succession and recruiting from inside. These enable the organization to respond to a rapidly changing environment and to minimize the time required for employing a new CEO.

Visible Results as Related to CEO Choice in Managing Work

Health care is a service that is difficult to measure. Profits are at best an ambiguous index of success. The data in this study suggest that

CEO effectiveness is perceived by trustees and medical staff leaders primarily in terms of the organization's achieving visible results. In response to the question, What are the key things he has done, good or bad, in his job? the chief of a clinical service at Washington Medical Center responds:

> . . . We have a large burn center. He put up the additional costs as an investment to see if it would work. . . . Long-range planning has been well thought out. . . . Managed care is being looked at. . . . He's always in on the appointment of professional people.

In response to the same question, a senior administrator at Van Buren Hospital answers:

> The biggest thing Larry did was the new building. . . . It took vision to apply for the OEO grant. . . . And we did the housing complex for the elderly. . . .

A senior administrator at Cleveland Hospital answers:

> Ted's built a new hospital. . . . There was a moratorium on capital projects. There was a series of technical reviews of the hospital's financial viability and debt feasibility that he had to go through for both hospital buildings which no one else had done.

The chief financial officer at Wilson HMO responds not in terms of building projects, but in terms of visible production and marketing activities:

> First, he made the [medical] groups full-time (he changed the delivery system). Second, he convinced the city government to buy the HMO package. . . . Third, [we expanded] into new regions and new markets with new products.

Constructing or renovating a building, expanding into a new region, obtaining a government grant, hiring a new chief of service, being ranked high among organizations in a national survey—these are all visible results. Less visible are such accomplishments as improving the technical quality of care and the amenities of service, promoting the career development of managers, and decreasing the unit cost of high-quality services for a given episode of illness. The less visible areas may be as important for organizational survival and growth, but they are not usually seen as equally important parameters for evaluating CEO effectiveness. They are therefore not areas that CEOs are likely to devote a great deal of time to managing. That situation may change if suitable measures of accomplishment are developed.

Although my observations and interviews indicate that CEOs commonly engage in less visible activities, these activities are mentioned less often by the CEOs and their associates. Interviewees were questioned specifically about CEO involvement in cost containment and quality assurance. The responses indicate that costs are being contained primarily through regular budgeting processes and in response to external regulatory controls. Standards relating to technical quality are increasingly being set and implemented, partly in response to state regulatory initiatives (particularly in the areas of physician credentialing, delineation of privileges, and review of physician work as indicated in the medical record). Another area of CEO involvement in quality, as indicated by the respondents, is the hiring and firing of clinical chiefs of service.

The following are examples of CEO participation in less visible areas:

—George:

> We control costs in the budget process, set realistic targets and monitor them. If revenues are lower because occupancy is lower, we try to alter the expense side to bring it closer. If you don't want to cut quality or standards, there comes a limit, unless you're going broke. What I've learned from bitter experience is that, once you cut personnel, you run the risk of a snowball effect. This is particularly true in nursing. The others quit—There's no way we can carry that load—and they can get a job somewhere else.

—Martin:

> [You must] create an environment in which others can have fun and use their imaginations. I'm good at these things. People here are not only smart, they're nice people and have remained at Van Buren a long time. I think their stability has been important to our neighborhood.

—Grover:

> Expense reduction is the result of constant management attention to unnecessary programs and staff caused by changes—you may no longer require certain things. . . . The future is another story, with managed care programs mandating less utilization; however, it's a short-term method at reduced expense per patient illness. It will not cap or reduce total expense levels over time. . . .

—Woodrow:

> On influencing the quality of service, we are undertaking several approaches. We are enhancing the amenities of our facilities, including upgrading the physical plans, interior design, equipment, and support systems. This is part of making the entire organization marketing-conscious. If you want people to have a positive image of themselves and their product, then you must give them adequate tools to work with.

Increasing Organizational Size and Complexity

The last crosscutting theme has to do with the increasing size and complexity of health care organizations and the implications for organizing the executive office. For example, Washington Medical Center is already a vast and complex institution with a mission of excellence in teaching, research, and service. Now it must consider as well the creation of affiliated networks for teaching and service and a response, with its medical staff and faculty, to managed care organizations. At the same time, it is attempting to raise funds and obtain approvals for a massive facility reconstruction program. Cleveland and Van Buren hospitals are discussing merger, and both are diversifying into areas other than inpatient medical care, such as ambulatory and long-term care. Wilson HMO is developing new products (IPAs and PPOs) and expanding into new regions. Both Wilson HMO and Cleveland Hospital have recently acquired other health care organizations through merger.

CEOs are spending a great deal of time outside their institutions. George observes:

> The CEO must be aware of the external environment and anticipate changes that must be made. . . . I have to be outside a good deal to sense what's going on in the environment and bring it back to the institution. . . . I spend one-third of my time outside the institution or on outside matters.

Martin worries about further expansion of Van Buren Hospital through merger and its effect on his job:

> What I fear about the merger situation is that the honeymoon is over in terms of what I've built here—I will have to set up new relationships and redefine the role of the institution. There's nothing in this but trouble for me. . . .

Grover sees his job as moving away from day-to-day management:

> My job is changing to become more policy-oriented. I spend more time outside the hospital on quality of care, malpractice, and reimbursement methodology. That produces problems back in the hospital and puts a lot of strain on me personally.

Woodrow would like to spend less time on day-to-day management; in his words:

> The pressures of overseeing a multistate health system are forcing changes in my present method of operations. The holding company will give me the opportunity to do that. It will force me to concentrate more fully on system-wide issues and new ventures.

In all four organizations, despite the presence of a chief operating officer, the CEO remains involved in operations and spends less time than three of the four desire or think appropriate on policy formulation and program development. Paradoxically, three of the four are said by some associates not to spend sufficient time on operations. On this point, a clinical chief at Cleveland Hospital (whose entire interview is not published here) observes with regard to Grover:

> The person at the top becomes divorced from day-to-day problems; he loses contact and loses his grip. Hospitals aren't used to this type of corporate structure. When I came here, there was more involvement in day-to-day problems than there is now. . . . He doesn't even know that acute episodes

are taking place. There are recurrent quality-of-care problems in certain services. He should be aware that the chiefs of certain services are not doing what they should about it.

Two of the CEOs say that they are hesitant to place COOs completely in charge of operations, either because the COOs are not fully trusted or because the CEOs are reluctant to yield responsibility. Woodrow, of Wilson HMO, comments:

> I must have confidence in the people I am delegating authority to, and the number of people I feel that confident about is limited. Experience, unfortunately, supports a cautious approach. At my previous job there were no more than three or four people I felt comfortable delegating broad responsibility to, and, given the size and diversity of this organization, I need to reach the point where I can have strong confidence in more people. Until that happens, I'll always be spread too thin.

In none of the four organizations does it appear that the COO is being groomed to eventually become CEO.

Recommendations to Managers

What I believe the data show is that, for these organizations and these CEOs, the health care industry is becoming more competitive. Further, the trustees and physician leaders in these organizations are seeing CEO performance as more critical to organizational survival and growth than it used to be. As yet, there is no measurable agreement on organizational goals or CEO contribution to goal attainment, nor is there any well-developed process for grooming successors. To the extent that there is local competition regarding price and quality and to the extent that the CEO is viewed as a critical contributor to the organization's obtaining or retaining market share, I would recommend the following:

1. Set and reset mutual expectations for organizational performance.
2. Develop the COO as the successor to the CEO.
3. Determine what skills and experience are required of the CEO.
4. Specify objectives for the CEO's contribution to organizational performance.

Set and Reset Mutual Expectations for Organizational Performance

Some of the objections to setting and resetting mutual expectations in large health care organizations include: (1) the difficulty of quantifying expectations (for example, what does "good patient care" mean?);

(2) conflicts of interest among managers, physicians, and trustees (for example, some hospital initiatives may threaten the revenues of certain attending physicians, or vice versa); (3) the cost and difficulty of reaching agreement on mutual expectations, especially when physicians and trustees are not being paid for their time; and (4) the lag time in resetting expectations in response to rapidly changing external pressures.

In response to these objections, I would argue that quantifying expectations may be difficult, but it is necessary. Even if expectations cannot be easily and acceptably quantified for all important aspects of organizational performance, there will be some aspects of behavior and performance that can be quantified. For example, Griffith (1987a) specifies several indicators of governing board performance in a community hospital, all of which can be quantified (see Figure 7.1).

Conflicts among constituencies and individuals in large health care organizations need to be recognized and dealt with in a common forum. This may result in the withdrawal from the organization of certain major players, notably physicians. I believe, however, that specifying goals will result in concentration of organizational effort, which, in turn, is likely to result in gain and retention of share in certain markets and appropriate withdrawal from others. Such concentration of effort is less likely to take place without goal specification.

I would argue that the benefits of having managers, physicians, and trustees spend time setting expectations outweigh the costs, that trustees should be chosen for their skill and experience in such activity, and that physicians and trustees should be paid for their time. Time spent formulating expectations can cut down on time spent gaining cooperation and thereby enhance the implementation of new initiatives.

Lag time between changing external pressures and agreement on expectations cannot be denied, but I would argue that time spent setting mutual expectations, including contingency planning, will result in enhanced ability to adapt to change. Line management, including physician managers, must be heavily involved in the planning process; it is too important to be left solely to staff planners.

Develop the COO as the Successor to the CEO

Some of the objections to planning managerial succession and developing the COO as the logical successor to the CEO in large health care organizations are (1) the CEO prefers the organization to remain as dependent upon his leadership as possible for the short term; (2) the best COO will not always be the best CEO; (3) planning CEO succession and COO development is costly in terms of time and conflict; and (4) other

Figure 7.1: Indicators of Governing Board Performance

Profitability
  Pricing
    Price comparability to competing institutions
    Price acceptability to third-party purchasers
    Price acceptability to patients
  Costs
    Comparative costs per episode of service (per discharge, per visit)
      Current values for this hospital and competing hospitals
      Percent change from preceding year
    Community costs per capita (costs per community member for hospital
      care)
      Current values for this community and similar communities
      Percent change from preceding year
  Profitability
    Bond rating
    Debt-equity ratio
    Funds available for capital and new programs
Access
  Changes in size and scope of service of this hospital and competing hospitals
Patient Satisfaction
  Hospital market share
    By community group (age, economic, ethnic, and so on)
    By kind of service (inpatient, outpatient, long-term, and so on)
  Satisfaction surveys (issues of costs, access, amenities, quality)
    Current patients
    Potential patients (community residents)
Donor Satisfaction
  Responses to fund drives
    Wealthy individual donors
    Corporate donors
    Community fund drives
Physician Satisfaction
  Number of doctors terminating privileges
    Transferring to other hospital
    Leaving community or retiring
  Number of doctors newly privileged in community
    This hospital
    Only at other hospitals
  Satisfaction reported by physicians
    Formal surveys
    Informal surveys
    Complaints received
Employee Satisfaction
  Vacancy statistics
  Turnover, grievance, and absenteeism statistics
  Employee satisfaction surveys

Source: Griffith (1987a, 186).

managers may leave the organization sooner than they would have if a successor had not been designated.

In response to these objections, I would argue that succession planning allows the CEO more choice in the selection of a successor and therefore increases the likelihood that the CEO's initiatives will be carried out. Also, many trustees and physician leaders prefer to know in advance whom they will be dealing with when the current CEO leaves.

To the objection that the person who is most effective as COO will not always be most effective as CEO, I would respond that the designated successor to the CEO should not always be the COO (although it is likely to be); it could be someone else in-house who will be formally developed for the job. If the designation and development process results in the departure of the COO or other key managers, it is probably better that they leave while the current CEO is effectively performing his job than when the CEO position is vacant or a new CEO has been appointed.

The designated successor to the CEO should be given the opportunity to learn, through visiting and reading, how similar organizations and their CEOs respond to the types of problems his or her organization faces. The successor should also begin to develop skills in areas in which he or she may be lacking—areas ranging from financial analysis to public speaking, from evaluating information systems to development of other managers.

Determine What Skills and Experience Are Required of the CEO

Why are organization-specific skills and experience not used as criteria for designating CEO successors or recruiting new CEOs? First, the trustees, who customarily select the CEO, may not themselves have the requisite skills and experience to evaluate a potential CEO. Second, the trustees may have limited experience with large health care organizations and therefore may not see that certain requirements of the CEO position are specific to their institution. Third, CEOs may be selected or designated for reasons other than their ability to do the job, for example, their personal attractiveness, reputation, or political connections with leading trustees or physicians.

I would point out that success as CEO of one large health care organization does not predict success as CEO of another large health care organization—each organization faces a different set of problems and a different political network. A primary consideration in selecting trustees of large health care organizations should be their experience and skill in evaluating and selecting CEOs. Other traditional functions of trustees can be carried out in other ways; for example, many hospitals have established a separate development organization. More trustees should be chief executives or trustees of other large health care organizations or of business organizations. Finally—and obviously—CEOs should be selected on the basis of their ability to do the job in a particular organization, at least so long as organizational growth and survival depend heavily on the CEO's contribution.

Specify Objectives for the CEO's Contribution to Organizational Performance

Some of the objections to specifying objectives for CEO contribution to organizational performance include: (1) there is no point in specifying CEO contribution if organizational objectives are not first specified; (2) CEO contribution may be more difficult to measure acceptably than organizational objectives; (3) the CEO, or the trustees, may prefer that the CEO's contribution *not* be specified, because they are satisfied with current organizational performance and CEO contribution—if it's not broken, don't fix it.

In response to these objections I would argue as follows: first, for reasons given previously, the organization should measure whether specific objectives have been attained within a given time and to what extent. CEO contribution may be more difficult to measure, but some important aspects of CEO work can be measured; one of these is the time spent and the results achieved on various projects and the appropriateness of this pattern of CEO time allocation relative to organizational objectives. (If trustees and the CEO specify objectives for the CEO's contribution, the CEO is likely to focus more on those objectives than on other concerns.) Many CEOs and trustees may prefer specification of CEO contribution, particularly when external pressures are changing rapidly and there is, without such specification, considerable disagreement among managers, physicians, and trustees on what the CEO should be doing and how. (I am assuming that the organization is not in crisis—in that case, there is little time for CEOs to do anything other than respond to the crisis.)

The trustees should evaluate and reward (or fail to reward) the CEO relative to his or her attainment of such objectives. This assumes appropriateness in the formulation of the objectives, provisions for changing objectives when internal or external circumstances require, and valid and reliable ways of measuring CEO contribution. (One way to measure such contribution is by analysis of activities and episodes of work, as discussed in Chapter 8.)

8.

Activities and Episodes of Work
as Evaluators of Performance

There are many ways of looking at what managers do; among them are roles, as developed by Mintzberg (1973, 54–99); functions of management, as introduced by Fayol (1949), Urwick (1952), and Carroll and Gillen (1987); and time studies, as performed by Mintzberg (1973) and Kurke and Aldrich (1983), among others.

I do not find Mintzberg's roles useful in evaluating what CEOs do. Roles are difficult to isolate and measure. In any one interaction, the CEO may be performing several roles simultaneously. How does the observer measure in a valid and reliable way the roles the CEO is performing when, for example, the CEO is watching a subordinate "manage"? Roles may be important for understanding what managers do, but they have not yet been transformed into effective units of measure.

I find Carroll and Gillen's functional approach to be more susceptible to valid and reliable measurement. Their managerial functions include staffing, planning, investigating, coordinating, evaluating, and supervising (Carroll and Gillen 1987). This approach is useful in categorizing managerial work, but Carroll and Gillen do not differentiate what is or is not such work; nor do they focus upon different episodes of work or projects, such as governance or community relations, which managers participate in regardless of function. I believe that episodes of work can be important in that respect—what episodes does the manager choose to manage? What results does he or she achieve? At what cost? Relative to what expectations?

I find Mintzberg's time analysis of managerial work useful, not in terms of assessing managerial effectiveness, but in assessing the skills and experience required for specific managerial positions. In connection with the skills and experience required of managers, my research validates Mintzberg's propositions, as abbreviated and shortened by Kurke and Aldrich. (Of Mintzberg's sample of CEOs, one of five was a hospital administrator; of Kurke and Aldrich's sample, one of four was.) The propositions (Kurke and Aldrich 1983) are as follows:

—Managers perform a great quantity of work with little time for breaks, and they must work beyond customary working hours.

—Managers' jobs are characterized by brevity, variety, and fragmentation.

—Managers clearly favor verbal over written contacts (that is, telephone calls and scheduled or nonscheduled meetings over desk work and tours).

—Scheduled meetings consume more of managers' time than any other activity.

—Managers spend little time in open-ended touring.

—Managers are boundary spanners, linking their organizations with the outside in a variety of ways. External contacts consume about half of the manager's verbal contact time.

—Subordinates generally consume about one-third to one-half of managers' total contact time.

—Managers spend relatively little time with superiors.

Kurke and Aldrich emphasize as well that daily routines leave little time for unscheduled meetings; when they do occur, they are short and almost always dyadic. Only in scheduled meetings do managers work in a group context. Only a minority of interpersonal contacts are self-initiated. Three-quarters of all contacts take place in the manager's office and take up two-fifths of contact time (Kurke and Aldrich 1983).

Consider Ted Grover's Monday, as shown in Table 8.1. This does not include any time Grover may have spent on work before or after coming to the office, nor did I ask Grover what he was thinking about during work. I did not ask what telephone calls he made or received or what he read during the hours before or after work. I count Grover as participating in 24 different activities and episodes of work during the Monday ob-

Table 8.1: Ted Grover's Episodes on a Monday

Episode with	Time Spent	Nature of Interaction for CEO
1. COO†	Brief	Is informed
2. COO †	Brief	Is informed
3. COO †	Brief	Is informed
4. Clinical chief	Brief	Is informed
5. COO †	Brief	Is informed
6. COO †	Brief	Requests information
7. COO †	Brief	Informs
8. COO †	Brief	Informs
9. COO †	Brief	Informs
10. COO †	Brief	Informs
11. COO †	Brief	Is informed
12. COO †	Brief	Informs
13. COO †	Brief	Informs
14. COO †	Brief	Informs
15. CEO of another hospital and consultant	Very long	Is informed, requests information, is asked for information
16. CFO	Brief	Is informed, requests information
17. COO††	Brief	Requests channeling after being informed
18. COO ††	Brief	Is informed
19. Trade association secretary	Brief	Informs
20. Secretary of medical disease organization	Brief	Informs
21. Secretary	Brief	Informs
22. CEO of another hospital	Brief	Informs
23. VP, medical affairs	Brief	Is informed
24. Assistant administrator	Brief	Is informed

Key: † means of hospital 1; †† means of hospital 2.

served. These ranged from a brief telephone call informing him that the vice-president for human resources had received a threat from a disgruntled worker, to two scheduled meetings of over seven hours regarding a possible merger.

Most of the brief activities lasted five minutes or less. Most of Grover's time, however, was spent on the scheduled meetings, not on desk work or tours (I kept no record of desk work in my log). Of the 24 brief contacts, 20 were with subordinates, four with outsiders, and none with board members. Most contacts were with subordinates, but most time was spent on external matters.

Of Grover's 24 brief interactions, all but 4 involved principally the sharing of information with internal managers. Regarding three of the other contacts, Grover requested information or was asked to supply information; in the last contact, he requested that donation proposals be channeled through the formal organizational structure.

These data are typical of all the days and all the CEOs I observed. To me, they support the model of the CEO in the large health care organization as "communicator, persuader, and shaper of organizational values and decisions" (Peters 1979, 170) rather than as problem solver and decision maker. The task of the CEO, according to Peters, is not "to impose an abstract order on an inherently disorderly process, but to become adept at the sorts of intervention by which he can nudge the organization in the desired direction and to some degree control its course" (page 172). This view runs counter to my own bias toward formulating objectives and measuring CEO performance on the basis of contribution to those objectives. The four organizations studied had never been subjected to any serious price competition that resulted in considerable numbers of patients' leaving one health care organization for another. I believe that, as such competition increases, more and more large health care organizations will specify objectives in order to retain and obtain market share.

Recommendations to Managers

Much of the general management literature focuses on functions of management, such as planning, coordinating, and controlling (Gulick 1937), or on the roles managers assume, such as negotiator, figurehead, or entrepreneur (Mintzberg 1973). As a result of following the four CEOs and parallel reading about episodes of illness as units of analysis in medical care (Strauss et al. 1985, 8–39; Hornbrook et al. 1985), I have become convinced that more attention should be paid, in evaluating CEOs and other managers, to analyzing their actual work rather than their roles and functions. This is particularly true insofar as managerial work relates to organizational objectives. Managerial activities can be categorized by subject. Episodes of work are clusters of activities on the same subject performed or participated in by the manager. Although this study was not designed to analyze activities or episodes of CEO work, I found, as the data were analyzed, that they emerged as a focus worthy of managerial consideration.

Episodes of work can be analyzed in terms of subject matter (who is involved in what kinds of interactions); whether the action requires CEO response, and if so, what kind of response; the CEO's choice of which episodes to manage and which to delegate or ignore; how much time the CEO chooses to devote to managing or participating in different episodes;

and results per managed episode versus costs in CEO time and other organizational resources.

Episodes of work can be used to analyze how the CEO is spending his or her time. This type of analysis can sharpen the CEO's focus on his or her behavior in relation to organizational objectives. It can also result in changes in or specification of organizational objectives when the CEO's time is being used effectively but not on current objectives.

Griffith points out that many of the activities a CEO performs are the normal "noise" of a working week. He suggests that an activity has a duration of two to four hours and that an episode has a duration of 1 to 24 months. "Things less than 20 minutes are noise, overhead, or something" (Griffith 1987b).

Implications for CEOs

If activities and episodes of work are such a good idea, why don't CEOs view their jobs in such terms, and why don't trustees evaluate CEOs in relation to patterns of episodes and results achieved relative to organizational objectives? Would there be any difference if these concepts were applied in large health care organizations? What are the costs of applying these concepts, and what is their validity and reliability in measuring CEO behavior? To what extent should CEO behavior be documented using that perspective? If the concepts are adopted, who should do the measuring? If CEO behavior is acceptable, why analyze it? Have the concepts of activities and episodes of work been successfully implemented anywhere? If so, with what results? These questions indicate limitations to the usefulness of these concepts. The limitations can be grouped into three categories: lack of standardized definitions, high costs of measurement; and limited rationale for such evaluation.

Lack of Standardized Definitions

Measurers are likely to disagree over what constitutes an activity or an episode. For example, how should different activities occurring in the same meeting be classified? Or the same activities occurring in different meetings? There is some question as to whether certain activities, constituting what Griffith refers to as noise or overhead, should be counted at all.

I agree that these limitations may be important for research in other than exploratory studies; however, I do not find them so significant as to outweigh the benefits of the concepts in analyzing CEO work. There are certain episodes of work that take up most of the CEO's time, or that should take up most of the time, relative to organizational objectives. CEOs should consider documenting what percentage of their time is being spent on what, what results they are accomplishing by episode, and how the pattern of results is and should be related to organizational objectives. I believe that documenting their work can significantly affect how CEOs decide to use their time and can thereby positively affect organizational performance.

High Costs of Measurement

A more serious limitation, I believe, is the perceived high cost of measuring activities and episodes. Activities will need to be coded by interactor, subject, disposition, and time spent, at least. To illustrate, the following are Tim George's first three activities on Monday (see Chapter 6):

1. Trustee requests the name of a doctor for a friend; CEO refers to COO (time spent: brief).
2. Other CEO calls indicating that his institution will not be part of a third organization's affiliation network for managed care (time spent: brief).
3. CEO participates with the dean in review of performance of a clinical chairman (time spent: intermediate).

These activities could be coded as follows:

1. Patient care request (PCR), from trustee X (T-X), brief time spent (B), referred to chief operating officer (REF-COO).
2. Managed care (MC), from chief executive officer Y (CEO-Y), brief time spent (B), information shared (INF).
3. Performance appraisal (PA), with dean re chief A (C-A), intermediate time spent (I), monitoring of fund raising (MON), dean must approve brochure (APP), must decide on space utilization re diabetes program and monitoring of outpatient surgery and resident program (DEC).

or, as follows:

Proposed CEO Worksheet

Item	Claimant	Time	Disposition
1. PCR	T-X	B	REF-COO
2. MC	CEO-Y	B	INF
3. PA	C-A	I	MON, APP, DEC

My assumption is that it will take the CEO no more than 15 to 30 extra minutes a day to keep track of his or her activities in this way. Recording (and having to explain the recording of) such activities while working will, however, increase strain. For example, the CEO must record talking on the telephone while talking (sometimes CEOs talk on two telephones almost at the same time), and CEOs are frequently interrupted. It assumes that the CEO will carry a recording pad and a pencil for documenting activities away from the office.

The log must be typed (and proofread for errors) and then the data grouped and analyzed. Activities can be grouped into episodes by an administrative assistant and reviewed by the CEO; however, the CEO may not wish to share how he or she spends time in such detail with anyone else. The time spent by the CEO on analysis will not be perceived as too long, I believe: it takes relatively little time for the CEO to read the data and decide whether he or she is spending enough time on organizational objectives or whether too much or too little time is being spent on certain episodes of work. What may take longer is analyzing how better to reallocate time or get better results for time spent, or whether to pursue changes in organizational objectives.

Limited Rationale

I am not suggesting that charting activities and episodes of work is necessary for effective management of large health care organizations; nor am I suggesting that effective managers of such organizations chart activities and episodes. I only suggest that the benefits of doing so may at times be significant. If there is no problem with organizational success or CEO performance, there may be no justification for such documentation. However, with today's increasing competition and turnover among CEOs, such charting and analysis will be beneficial to many of them as documentation of what they do; as an aid to formulation of more realistic organizational objectives; and as an aid to better allocation of their time at work.

Documenting what the CEO does. A record of what the CEO said to whom when may be useful in future conversations regarding claims and promises. The CEO will be able to share what he or she does with evaluators, peers, and subordinates. It is useful for CEOs to be able to explain what they do, compare their work with that of other CEOs in like positions, and compare CEO work with that done by subordinates, in order to better organize work.

Given that many health care organizations are not-for-profit and that many of their trustees are not selected for proven ability to make policy decisions for such organizations, charting and analysis of CEO time by episode of work will be useful in orienting trustees to what the CEO does.

Formulating organizational objectives. Comparing what the CEO does with what the organization is supposed to be accomplishing can be useful whether the two are in alignment or not. If alignment is good, the CEO and those who evaluate the CEO have the documentation to validate it. If the alignment is off, analysis can reveal either that the CEO is not spending time as appropriately as he or she should or that the organization's objectives are not sufficiently specific, feasible, or desirable. Assuming the latter to be the case, trustees and managers may spend time specifying more useful organizational objectives.

Allocating the CEO's time. For the CEO, there are two effects of charting and analyzing time: (1) reallocation of time based upon analysis of past patterns and (2) reallocation of time to conform to the expectations of whoever holds the CEO formally accountable for how his or her time is spent. Perhaps one of the perquisites of CEOs has been not having to account for their time by episodes of work, but I question whether this is in the best interests of the organization and of those who pay for care and supply the organization with resources.

In practice, a CEO may implement such a charting and analysis system for his or her sole use during the first month or two, in order to overcome problems in implementation, refine the charting system, and evaluate benefits relative to costs. During a trial period the CEO and others can evaluate whether changes toward more complete documentation seem advisable.

Implications for Teaching Management

Criteria for graduate curricula in health services administration established by the Accrediting Commission on Education for Health Services Administration (1982) do not include any emphasis on the work managers do.

In three commonly used health services management textbooks—namely, *Health Care Management,* edited by Shortell and Kaluzny (1983); *Management of Health Services,* edited by Kaluzny et al. (1982); and *Managing Health Services Organizations,* edited by Rakich, Longest, and Darr (1985)—there is no mention of episodes of work or time management in the index. In programs in health care management education this material may be covered in courses on organizational behavior or management—or it may be assumed that managers should learn this on the job rather than in school.

A few articles have been written about how managers of health care services spend their time. In a paper on hospital administrators and organizational effectiveness published in 1972, I cited studies of how administrators spend their time in a university teaching hospital (Connors and Hutt 1967) and in 55 Catholic and non-Catholic hospitals (Murray et al. 1968). In both studies, the authors measured time spent in the following functions: planning, directing and coordinating, extramural, personal, controlling, organizing, and operating. The subject seems to be of less interest currently. For example, scanning the last three years of *Hospital and Health Services Administration* and *Health Care Management Review,* two popular health services management journals, I can find no titles of articles on this subject. Neuhauser and I did not come across any articles on this subject when working on our textbooks of readings (1987) and case studies (1986) on health services management.

There is a relevant case study on time management—an in-basket exercise by E. Paul Smith (1983). In this exercise, an assistant administrator is given a pile of 21 items (or episodes of work) and is told to (1) list each of the items in the in-basket, (2) assign a priority to each item, (3) indicate what action he or she would take, and (4) identify who should be responsible for each item (that is, to whom he or she should delegate it). The assistant administrator is also asked to list any general problems he or she believes might exist within the hospital and the rationale for citing them.

This is not the place to discuss what part analysis of activities and episodes of work plays in the health care management education curriculum. Students and professors have told me how effective it is when managers share their actual in-basket with students and ask them what they would do with particular problems or opportunities. I do believe it is particularly useful if persons lacking experience in health care organizations or in management can be shown how managers spend their time and on what, what results managers get from various kinds of interventions, and how these results contribute to organizational effectiveness. It is important for faculty members who teach organizational sociology and behavior and management courses to know what managers do.

Not knowing what managers do can result in naiveté or cynicism. Either can have a negative effect on the performance of inexperienced managers by clouding their understanding of the constraints and opportunities faced by themselves, their bosses, and their peers. I believe that lack of knowledge about managerial work presents a greater danger to inexperienced managers than lack of knowledge about most of the things they are currently taught in required graduate and undergraduate courses. How information about what managers do should be learned depends upon the source materials available and upon faculty who are capable of and interested in this kind of teaching.

Implications for Management Research

Neuhauser suggests projects (rather than episodes) as the appropriate unit of analysis for managerial work (1987). Projects have a clear beginning when they come to the manager's attention. There follows a sequence of activities, and sometimes there is a clear ending. Examples of managerial projects include obtaining a certificate of need, starting a new service, building, recruiting a senior manager or physician, and organizing an important meeting.

Neuhauser raises the following research questions about project management:

—What percent of the manager's time is spent this way? Some activities, such as reading mail or walking around the hospital, would not qualify. Projects may need to be further defined by duration, those which last more or less than one week.

—What is the average number of projects that a manager actively carries? What is the range? What is the optimal number? Too few projects or too many probably signifies ineffectiveness.

—Are different projects carried out with different management styles? Is this a useful question to ask?

—What are important descriptors of projects? Some descriptors are duration, managerial time required, time horizon for financial payoff, number of persons involved, and amount of financial resources involved.

—How does the manager decide when the project has ended? How many do end? How does the manager decide if the outcome is successful?

—How do these projects fit with the strategic plan and corporate mission? Do they articulate well? Can the projects be scored for such relevance?

Neuhauser then presents variables related to the manager, to the hospital, and to the project. Variables related to the manager include perceived competence, level in the organization, managerial experience, number of projects underway, percent completed, percent completed successfully. Variables related to the hospital include size and complexity. Variables related to the project include duration, managerial time required, endpoint or no endpoint, level of success, closeness of relationship to organizational objectives, management style used, number of people involved, and projected relationship to constituency group (such as medical staff or governing board). Neuhauser suggests that factor, or cluster, analysis can be used to group these descriptors. With a well-defined dependent variable such as level of project success, regression analysis can be used (Neuhauser 1987).

I find "project" a less useful term than "episode," because most projects in large health care organizations are not solely or primarily managerial. They may involve clinicians or even managers of other organizations who are managing their own episodes of work as part of the project. Episodes focus more on managerial than group accomplishment and include more short-term and investment activities, such as activities in support of other managers. (Such support activities can also be called projects, so this may be a matter of semantic preference.)

Research is needed on what effects the charting and analyzing of activities and episodes of work will have on the allocation of a CEO's time and on the closeness of the relationship between CEO allocation of time by episode on specific organizational objectives. One would expect analysis to have a greater effect on contributions to the extent that the CEO is formally evaluated by others and to the extent that such analysis is used as part of the CEO's evaluation. I would expect analysis of work episodes to result in a reallocation of CEO time toward more specific organizational objectives, depending upon type of health care organization, circumstances, and the CEO's skills and experience.

Research is also needed on the validity and reliability of activities and episodes as measures of managerial work. I do not claim any special expertise in this area; I only wish to draw attention to the importance of developing a common language and system of measurement among researchers and managers, including physician leaders.

I agree with Hales that the concept of managerial effectiveness depends on managerial performance relative to expectations, and that such expectations are held by those who formally evaluate the manager or upon whose sufferance the manager's job depends (Hales 1986). It would be interesting, therefore, to relate tenure and pay raises to variance between the CEO's expectations regarding his or her performance and the expectations of the CEO's evaluators. A small or positive variance would predict longer tenure and higher raises in pay; a large or negative variance would predict the opposite.

A Final Word

Finally, what is the usefulness of this book? First, it provides information to health care managers and others regarding what CEOs do in these organizations. This should increase understanding of the role of managers in health care organizations and be useful to those who want to become managers and CEOs in these organizations. Second, it focuses attention on the importance of specifying objectives in health care organizations that are measurable and of viewing CEO work in terms of activities and episodes of work and relating the two. I suggest this as a possible approach to evaluating the effectiveness of health care organizations and of managers who are accountable in an important way for their effectiveness. Hopefully, this approach will be of use to those who practice health care management, teach it, and do research on it. If I have come up with no definitive answers to what makes CEOs of large health care organizations effective in their jobs, I believe I have raised useful questions in determining such effectiveness. What are the measurable objectives of the organization? How does the CEO spend his or her time? What are the expectations of those who evaluate the CEO concerning CEO contribution to attainment of organizational objectives? If there is considerable divergence between specified organizational objectives and how the CEO spends time, should one or the other be changed? If organizational objectives are not specified in measurable ways, nor management time accounted for, what is the effect on organizational survival and retention of market share? And the effect on managerial job security and compensation? And what should be the effect?

References

Accrediting Commission in Education for Health Services Administration. 1982. *Criteria for a Graduate Program in Health Services Administration*. Washington, D.C.: ACEHSA.

Brown, Lawrence D. 1983. *Politics and Health Care Organization: HMOs as Federal Policy.* Washington, D.C.: The Brookings Institution.

Carroll, Stephen J., and Dennis J. Gillen. 1987. Are the Classical Management Functions Useful in Describing Managerial Work? *Academy of Management Review* 12: 38–51.

Connors, Edward J., and Joseph C. Hutt. 1967. How Administrators Spend Their Day. *Hospitals* 41: 45ff.

Fayol, Henri. 1949. *General and Industrial Management,* trans. C. Storrs. London: Pitman.

Fiedler, Fred E. 1964. A Contingency Model of Leadership Effectiveness. In *Advances in Experimental Social Psychology,* ed. Leonard Berkowitz, 149–90. New York: Academic Press.

——. 1971. Validation and Extension of the Contingency Model of Leadership Effectiveness: A Review of Empirical Findings. *Psychological Bulletin* 76: 128–48.

Griffith, John R. 1987a. *The Well-Managed Community Hospital.* Ann Arbor: Health Administration Press.

——. 1987b. Personal communication.

Gulick, Luther. 1937. Notes on a Theory of Organization. In *Papers on the Science of Administration,* eds. Luther Gulick and Lyndall Urwick, 3–13. New York: Institute of Public Administration.

Hales, Colin P. 1986. What Do Managers Do? A Critical Review of the Evidence. *Journal of Management Studies* 23 (1): 88–115.

Hornbrook, Mark C., Arnold V. Hurtado, and Richard E. Johnson. 1985. Health Care Episodes: Definition, Management, and Use. *Medical Care Review* 42: 163–218.

Kaluzny, Arnold D., D. Michael Warner, David G. Warren, and William N. Zelman, eds. 1982. *Management of Health Services.* Englewood Cliffs, N.J.: Prentice-Hall.

Kotter, John P. 1985. *Power and Influence.* New York: Free Press.

Kovner, Anthony R. 1972. The Hospital Administrator and Organizational Effectiveness. In *Organization Research on Health Institutions,* ed. Basil S. Georgopoulos, 355–76. Ann Arbor: University of Michigan.

————. 1985. Improving the Effectiveness of Hospital Governing Boards. *Frontiers of Health Services Management* 2 (1): 4–33.

Kovner, Anthony R., and Martin Chin. 1985. Physician Leadership in Hospital Strategic Decision Making. *Hospital & Health Services Administration* 30 (6): 64–79.

Kovner, Anthony R., and Duncan Neuhauser, eds. 1986. *Health Services Management: A Book of Cases,* 2d ed. Ann Arbor: Health Administration Press.

————. 1987. *Health Services Management: Readings and Commentary,* 3d ed. Ann Arbor: Health Administration Press.

Kurke, Lance B., and Howard E. Aldrich. 1983. Mintzberg Was Right! A Replication and Extension of the Nature of Managerial Work. *Management Science* 29: 975–84.

Levinson, Harry, and Stuart Rosenthal. 1984. *CEO, Corporate Leadership in Action.* New York: Basic Books.

Lopez, Barry. 1986. *Arctic Dreams.* New York: Scribner's, pp. 95–96.

Mintzberg, Henry. 1973. *The Nature of Managerial Work.* New York: Harper & Row.

Murray, Ralph T., Paul R. Donnelly, and Margaret Threadgold. 1968. How Administrators Spend Their Time: A Research Report. *Hospital Progress* 49: 49–58.

Neuhauser, Duncan. 1987. Personal communication.

Peters, Thomas J. 1979. Leadership: Sad Facts and Silver Linings. *Harvard Business Review* 79: 164–72.

Rakich, Jonathan S., Beaufort Longest, and Kurt Darr, eds. 1985. *Managing Health Services Organizations.* Philadelphia: Saunders.

Shortell, Stephen M., and Arnold D. Kaluzny, eds. 1983. *Health Care Management.* New York: Wiley.

Smith, E. Paul. 1983. Unity Hospital (An In-Basket Exercise). In *Cases in Health Services Management,* eds. Jonathan Rakich et al., 207–18. Philadelphia: Saunders.

Strauss, Anselm, Shizuko Fagerbaugh, Barbara Suczek, and Carolyn Wiener. 1985. *Social Organization of Medical Work.* Chicago: University of Chicago Press.

Urwick, Lyndell F. 1952. *Notes on the Theory of Organization.* New York: American Management Association.

Further Reading

Cohen, Michael D., and James A. March. 1986. *Leadership and Ambiguity,* 2d ed. Boston: Harvard Business School.

Duby, Georges, and William Marshal. 1985. *The Flower of Chivalry.* New York: Pantheon.

Himmelstein, David U., and Steffie Woolhandler. 1986. Cost Without Benefit: Administrative Waste in U.S. Health Care. *New England Journal of Medicine* 314: 441–44.

Katz, Robert L. 1974. Skills of an Effective Administrator. *Harvard Business Review* September-October: 90–102.

Komaki, Judith L. 1986. Toward Effective Supervision: An Operant Analysis and Comparison of Managers at Work. *Journal of Applied Psychology* 71: 270–79.

Kotter, John P. 1982. *The General Managers.* New York: Free Press.

Mintzberg, Henry. 1983. *Power in and Around Organizations.* Englewood Cliffs, N.J.: Prentice-Hall, pp. 119–26.

Stewart, Rosemary. 1982. *Choices for the Manager.* Englewood Cliffs, N.J.: Prentice-Hall.

Appendix A

Questions Asked During Interviews with CEOs

First Interview

1. When you took over as CEO, what strong wishes, thoughts, aspirations, ambitions did you have in mind?
2. When you were selected for your CEO tasks, were you given a specific charge by the board? Did that charge differ significantly from what you yourself saw had to be done? What did you hope to be able to do beyond the expectations of the board?
3. What did you see had to be done in and to the organization in order to achieve those goals? That is, what policies, practices, perceptions, methods, attitudes did you perceive had to be changed?
4. How did you go about changing policies, practices, perceptions, methods, and attitudes?

5. Looking back on it now, how well did you succeed in making those changes? Did they produce the effects you were striving for? How do you know?

6. Describe your job. Being very effective in the job means what?

7. What were the toughest decisions you have had to make as a manager?

8. If you were to point out one or more major pitfalls for persons in your job, what would they be?

9. When you want to leave your organization, what managerial changes do you want to leave behind? That is, what will indicate that you have had an enduring effect on your organization?

10. Who among your peers has done something in his or her organization that you wish you had been able to do in yours? Why can't you do it?

11. What stories do people tell about you?

Second Interview

1. What makes for an effective manager in your organization?

2. How are you evaluated? By whom? How do you evaluate yourself?

3. What are the barriers to managing effectively in your organization, and how do you overcome them?

4. What are the opportunities for managing effectively in your organization, and how do you take advantage of them?

5. To what extent are you an effective manager? How can you be more effective?

6. How did you learn to be an effective manager in this organization? What have you learned?

7. What is your agenda for the short term? For the long term?

8. How will you accomplish these? Through what networks?

9. How is your job changing?

10. How is your job performance changing?

11. How do you influence the cost of medical care in your organization? Give examples.

12. In what ways do internal and external groups affect your ability to influence costs and the ways in which you influence costs?

13. Why don't you do more to control costs in this organization?

14. How do you influence the quality of medical care in this organization? Give examples.

15. In what ways do external and internal groups affect your ability to influence quality and the ways in which you influence quality?

16. Why don't you do more to assure quality in this organization?

17. Are there any comments or thoughts you would like to share relevant to this study with regulators, other managers, educators, or researchers?

Appendix B

Questions Asked During Interviews with CEOs' Associates

1. What is your background? How long and where have you worked with the manager? What are those problems or issues on which you have worked most closely with the manager?
2. What are the key things one needs to understand about this business and this organization in order to truly understand the context in which the general manager works?
3. What are the key things he has done, good or bad, in his job? Why did he do them? What impact did they have?
4. How do you normally interact with him? When and for how long? How does he get things done? What is he trying to do? What are the sources of his power?
5. How would you describe him as a manager? As a person?
6. How would you rate his performance? Why?

7. In what ways has he changed the way he manages or what he manages? Why?
8. What stories do people tell about him?
9. How does he influence the cost of medical care in your organization? Give examples.
10. How does he influence the quality of medical care in your organization? Give examples.

About the Author

ANTHONY R. KOVNER, M.P.A., Ph.D., is currently Director, Program in Health Policy and Management, and Professor, School of Public Administration, at New York University. He also serves as Senior Program Consultant to the Robert Wood Johnson Foundation and is Director of the Foundation's Hospital-Based Program to Improve Rural Health Care. Dr. Kovner is a member of the Board of Trustees of Lutheran Medical Center and Augustana Nursing Home in Brooklyn, New York. Before joining NYU, he was Chief Executive Officer of the Newcomb Hospital of Vineland, New Jersey, and Senior Health Consultant to the United Autoworkers Union in Detroit, Michigan. He is the author of *Really Trying: A Career Guide for the Health Services Manager.*